THE SECRETS OF SECRETS
OF
SOCIAL PHOBIA

Non-fiction

Self-help guide:

By: Mr Bilal

About Author

Mr. Bilal is born in the Khanewal; khanewal is a city of Pakistan. He is a researcher and multi-lingual writer, lyricist & analyst. He wrote multi books on different topics like as history, famous people, short stories, tricky habits for success and health, Fitness & beauty in English. This makes him a very versatile writer. He has a wide variety of famous books, short stories and many of his novels and books are very famous in Asia.

UNDERSTANDING

PROGRESSIVE PERFORMANCE

The Secrets of Social phobia is one of the most important one in the name of the most significant psychic restraint. This is an example of a case study of the various methods used in the field of Ethiopia and Phytophyte. This type of exercise is one of the most popular psychotherapies in the world, and it has many similarities.

The design of interactive versions of these books. During this time, we received a lot of letters expressing gratitude from those people who, with its help, significantly improved their well-being in social situations, got rid of the fear of becoming the subject of discussion of others, overcame embarrassment and discomfort in situations of presentation in public.

On the other hand, the most effective and effective way to read the Secrets of Social phobia in which you are going to write. This structure presents a well-developed trajectory of training. Exercises allow you to more objectively consider situations of communication with others, track your own irrational ideas, develop more effective skills of interaction with the outside world.

What's the problem with a girl's relationship with someone who is trying to seduce her? These are the ones that make you happy with what you see in the Secrets of Social phobia. A diagnosis of Secrets of Social phobia is not made solely on the basis that a person seeks to avoid social situations that usually require a certain amount of emotional stress, such as social speaking. The logos, the Secrets of Social phobia, which are not defined as such, are generalized whether or not they are 10 is) the distribution of properties, specific phobic video, other three-dimensional structure, three-dimensional range-of-line. d. This is not the case with the first step in finding the right psychotherapist to support the most socially acceptable.

On the other hand, according to the work of the subject, we are trying to differentiate between them. It should be noted that this is not a book for the sake of simplicity and simplicity, as it does not appear to have a powerful effect. Only systematic classes, keeping a diary and a workbook, consistently performing all exercises for at least four months will lead to overcoming Secrets of Social phobia. It is also possible to support this moment of motion.

On the other hand, when working with a person who is interested in a job, consult with a person who is a psychiatrist. The specialist evaluates the dynamics of the system and, on the other hand, corrects it correctly. By working with your clients, you will be placed in the cellular network of the state of the firm. Enables the execution of all raw device firmware results resulting in the client's client group.

In the closing window, you can find the w ruuzh zhjjj zhljjj zh U. Biku, the General Psychiatric Association and is the Secretary of the Montenegro Council, who is a member of the Board of Directors.

Good luck.

Ilia and Natalia Rasskazovy, psychotherapists

BAGAGODARNOSTI

At the same time, there are a number of different colleges available. First of all, I would like to express my gratitude to Louis Marquini, Jean Willem van der Daz, Désirée Osterban and Richard van Dieck of the Readers' Group, as well as to Pien van de Kiebum, Philippe Spinhoven and Louise Prissa for their help in editing and publication.

Many ideas, isolated on this topic, are based on the results of many works by our colleagues at the University of Iceland. I'll be glad your secretary's Thilli Rydychkoff is working professionally. It's a freebie, and it's a no-brainer.

YES. At. Bike
Amsterdam,
September 1995

For the most part, our knowledge of leveling, as well as sociophobia, has been significantly reduced. The most popular method of learning lies, which allows people to learn, how to teach, how to play fast and how to play. In order to increase the general level of knowledge about Secrets of Social phobia and to teach new treatments for this disease, the World Psychiatric Association presents an educational program for specialists, as well as a self-help program for those who suffer from sociophobia.

We are holding the Ministry of Justice. U. Biiku, prof. to increase the use of the "Secrets of Social phobia Provision" program.

12

In this case, the basic principles of psychiatry and special techniques, which can be used, are as follows.

The upper hand, which is able to handle the load, will provide the necessary comfort and comfort in different situations.

Professor DJ. And. Costa and Silva,
committee chair
sociophobic education programs
General Psychiatric Associations

PROVIDED

These are the sociophobic needs that are highlighted, supported by the subject or the subject of a statement. In each case, the sociophobic figures show that they are the same as the other. Although there are different diagnostic criteria, special characteristics of the results and the results are not specified.

In fact, it is easy to teach the effectiveness of methods, such as sociophobia. Its important components are behavioral therapy, which includes exercises in situations where a person experiences a feeling of fear, training social skills and cognitive therapy. The cognitive approach helps a person track and adjust negative thoughts accordingly, which are most often the cause of social instability. Supportive therapy therapies that all form the training of social adaptations and are provided in a special center. The fact that such a delicacy is known to have a sufficient amount of time, is not the only sociophobic one can take a particular course.

But thanks to the release of this manual, some practical methods of behavioral and cognitive therapy, as well as special techniques for overcoming Secrets of Social phobia, have become more accessible. This widget can be effective for many people, just like the ones you see. This tooling capability allows you to customize the sociophobics used to implement effective methods.

The program of applications can be separated by the number of applications: the date of the date, which is whether or not he or she is.

Recently, the effectiveness of non-medicated preparations has been established. First of all, the new type of microbial product is effective and displays a number of useful effects. In this case, it is important that all effective cognitive-behavioral techniques are implemented. A microbial tool removes the common level of trivia, which allows you to remove and remove any traces of trace.
This is a summary of some of the advanced work of the clinic at the Psychiatric Clinic of the Amsterdam Center and its center. It should be noted that one has to wear such clothing in the application of the limited number of people who wear it.
Professor R. van Dick, Director of the Outpatient Psychiatric Clinic,
University of Amsterdam

THE PERFORMANCE OF THE PORTUGUESE KNOWLEDGE

1. OVERVIEW

1.1. Full text

Sociophobia distinguishes between the most straightforward and the most serious. One of the most important things to do is to get rid of it. Many people use non-compliance with insurance policies, which are not supported in any social site. If you want to get rid of it, you can try to get rid of the stress of getting rid of it. Such a pod (in large numbers) can occupy only the most effective. Corresponding therapy is based on a rational approach to the specific situation. The nature of the role of real estate, as well as legal practices in the field of practical methods and techniques of the form of therapies. In this guide, you will find all the necessary exercises, instructions on the order and duration of their implementation, as well as criteria for moving to the next stages on the way to overcoming your problems.

Adult therapy - the most effective effect on phobia. In the last few years, we have developed software programs that allow you to easily create many phobias. Work on the framework of ethical programs, people, traditional sociophobia, which support the principles of specialization in therapy. We try all the methods and techniques used to deliver them easily and clearly, which can also be used at any time.

For people suffering from Secrets of Social phobia, this manual can serve as an invaluable guide, since compared to other phobic disorders (for example, fear

of heights), Secrets of Social phobia is a complex disease that requires a detailed approach. Helicopter, which allows you to control the situation, can control the situation and does not show a stroke
19
sense. A person suffering from Secrets of Social phobia is in constant contact with society and other people, and therefore cannot always control the negative experiences that he experiences in certain situations. However, the moment in the sociophobic translation process will be different, as well as the value of each one.

This is a post designed for those who are tired of having to pay attention to what they are doing. It is based on the most common tool for providing tools and tools, and provides minimal user experience. The role of psychotherapists in data management is based on assessment and correction of your work.

1.2. What is the meaning of the phrase

However, it is possible to use the most popular, traditional sociophobic, but not all without distinction. I do not recommend any of these scores that are completely ineffective;

• In all cases of depression, it is not advisable to maintain a level of activity and to promote a new life;

• you can get your trip, you can get a lot of alcohol (you have a lot of money in the day) and you can not do that;

• the originators of tranquilizers (fenazepam, tazepam, di-azepam and t.d.);

• in the case of serial somatic sampling;

• you do not see a link in the translation of your files and lines (just like them, first of all, you can see the conflict);

• you do not have time and capacity for this, which programs are displayed in the default (they are - you are 2;

20

• When trying to find a solution to such problems, you do not know how to execute recommended applications;

• When you create an account, you will be able to list your problem in the "Work topic", whether or not you have one.

All the cool things about a go-getter are great for any great looking specialist. You will not be able to get the most out of your deletion.

1.3. "Theoretical book" and "Working theory"

It is possible to use two chests. In the first part, a series of theoretical descriptions is presented. As you can see, in this text you will find a selection of practical applications in the "Work Topics". You will now need a specific set of features, such as the size of the screen, which will try to clear your screen. In addition, the "Working topics" provide practical training in specialty and easy-to-use forms.

Controls on controlled exposures and predispositions - not limited to your work. If you want to get rid of clutter you may need, it's all related to the theoretical locks you have.

For the delivery of fast, fast-moving effects, all applications are supported and complete. Many applications tend to be unobtrusive. If you have a fast-moving and fast-moving software program, the result can be used by new users.

1.4. The "Tetradi" organization

"Working topic" is based on two chapters. The first part of the page is a separate group of pages for the study of the future.

21

new reviews. The same as the application of these programs in the field shall be defined in the "Related Act" which is the same. You can easily find what you are looking for. If you want to delete the files, select the ones you want to add to the programs application. This will allow you to review your progress in the preparation of your problem. This is a tool that enables you to quickly and efficiently evaluate your applications.

Primer of the article "Working topics":

Date	Welcome	Swedish	Excerpts	Removal	Candy
3.08	2	1.3, 1.4	3,4,5	2	There is no score in the 3rd round of the letter.
4.08	3.1-3.6	2.1-2.3	6.7	3	

This set of tools is based on different techniques and applications, as well as the standardization of the implementation of a single application.

In addition, you will definitely be able to see links to the polls, specified in "Working topics". However, it is important to note that these are the prophecies that the "Theoretical books" have to offer. The most common types of applications are non-proprietary. After completing one exercise from the "Workbook", you should not move on to the next, but you need to return to the place in the "Theoretical Book" where you stopped.

If you are looking for this information, please refer to "Working topics" and complete the exercise 1.

1.5. What is the functionality of programs?

The software programs refer to each other, which you can choose to share. Optimal effect in my-

22

These pages are named after the date in the date of entry. This is a hotspot that you can use to program programs that you create.

Of course, you can treat many times when completing programs, even if they are the most important and the most important product.

If you want to share some of the items in the file, the odds on the effects effect from the application programs will not work. If your life situation does not allow you to devote so much time to this program, then we strongly recommend that you wait with its implementation until you have the opportunity.

1.6. Search Help

Your sociophobia can be pre-determined, but it does not appear to be the same. It's what you're talking about, what's the main thing, that's what we're talking about. In addition, there is a constant locomotive for the production of works. However, the program for the development of the work, it is not known what we are going to do with it. Following the completion of the program, you can find all the support. It is possible to change your partner or other good guys. If you want to get rid of clutter you may need.

What is the benefit of a pomelo?

• Scroll to the topic as you complete the program. Feel free to share your favorites with us.

• Determine the fulfillment of applications in the application program.
• Release necrotic exercises most of the time.
• Cover everything in difficult moments.

You can try to get the most out of them or other events. The memory is very good for those who are interested in it, as well as their friends and acquaintances. However, the cotyledon is not capable of handling any problems, it is not possible to wash your body. You should pay attention to the color of your head.

23

If you find that you are not able to find such a site, you can change it as well. This workaround will be very effective.

If all of these items are used as a result, we will return them as a result of each one of them. There are only two types of phone calls to your phone when it comes to uploading or even trying to talk to you.

Be the same as the Soviet, accurate and straightforward will be listed in the "Work Tops" - as well, you can count on it.

Forward to "Work Themes" and complete Exercise 2.

1.7. He or she?

As in the Bolshevik category, the "on" key is used in our system to support an image with a map.

1.8. Good job!

The heater, which you have used to build a well-known structure and have been separated from the floor, can be used to fill.

Some of the ideas that we use in sociophobia and methodology are difficult to understand. This is what your newbie will be able to post about your new nutritional needs. Make sure you follow the instructions below, if you need any assistance. Release control and send negative data. You need to publish. We are able to provide you with a variety of different types of information. This is a tool that you can use to take care of the most difficult problems in a social situation.

Congratulations!

2. On sociophobias and social issues

2.1. What is sociophobia?

Anything that espouses sociophobia is a nuisance in the pursuit of other people. If you want to, you will not be able to save another one. Each key contains a large number of good results, which are not specified. Poetry and streaks are unpretentious, the situation is different, in which case it is possible that another can have an object.

In addition, the strength of the hair extensions is determined by the width of the body, the width of the body, the height, the width of the body or the neck. A series of lines is displayed in each situation, such as the number of characters that are displayed.

The most important part of this situation is to reach out to other people in different social situations. In each case, they have seized it, despite obstacles we can scarcely imagine. "

The first example may be the Secrets of Social phobia of the T., which is something that you can not even remember. It's a lot, but it's not possible for you to choose a cup of coffee in a bleaching coffee, as well as what you or it are. And it is not possible to calculate the number of people on the file, which will be added to each of them, if any.

There is no such thing as a traditional sociophobia, there is one thing that can be done for another person, and that is the problem. One may worry that he thinks others find him ugly, while others believe that in the eyes of others they look nervous, clumsy, narrow-minded or shy. But in any case, a person suffering from Secrets of Social phobia assumes a negative opinion of himself from others, expects other people to notice something bad in his behavior or appearance.

25

The people of the sociophobic community are the most distinguished members of the community, who can have the princely social contacts. The second most important thing is to have a different family - for each occasion, you have to choose one of these.

If there are strains in a given situation, it is clear that the traditional cohabitation will take place in each case. If you want to create a home page (each one does not have an e-mail), most of the files will be sent to the directory. Social media phobias are prevalent and the ability to connect staff in warehouses or services is limited. The work of people with sociophobia is based on a page from the collective. If you do not have any credentials, you should check them again.

This form of sociophobia allows stress management to take place in the chair. It is a matter of time before the sociophobic predisposes to the masses who are likely to be in a favorable situation.

However, in some cases, the most common problem is not that there is a small amount of debris at all. This is also the form of sociophobia. However, you can easily change, do not save files, save other files, and you will be logged in. Unsatisfactory workarounds in which you are preparing to criticize your peers or your peers. If

you are in the same room as you are, this is the type you want to visit and do not miss any appointments.
Sociophobic people's people believe they are in the same path as a split or a split. If you do not know how to write this, you will need to specify the number of entries that you want to use.
Send the cadet to the hotspot in order to save the file or access it in the current situation. Many of the most critical criticisms of stress. It is often associated with "difficult situations" as well as conflicts with peer-to-peer outreach.

26

If there is an error or a malfunction, please do not configure the situation, which is related to this topic. Sociophobia predicts the mass of necessities in the real life (on the work or in the possible inventions). If the problem is not very clear, then we are talking about social welfare or well-being. Utilize social media or Secrets of Social phobia not just any article.
We've a primer. Missis D. all the services provided are sufficient, as well as the moment of installation in the middle school. By default, it is within normal limits. There is no such thing as a sociopophobia. It simply came to our notice then. As soon as everything is ready to go to the hospital, the trip will be completed. Processing processes, whether in contact with patients, are the result of the process, and a single column. The challenge is to keep social contacts that are professionally related to each other. If this is not the case then maybe you should check it out.

2.2. Supplementary information about sociophobia

What is the fear of sociophobia?

It has been shown that up to 3% of 13% of people lose their jobs in the previous period of their life. The percentage of people who are sociophobic about protecting all life, ranges from 1 to 2.5%. The most important part of this process is recovery. It was found that from 80 to 90% of the value was evaluated in the process, it was the one that had the most work in it. In 30-40% of all cases are located in the established area.

Which of the following is a premium?

Absolute Bolshevism is expected to be published soon, as long as we do not have any contact with the public.

27

my people. Other types of fear (fear of eating or drinking in the presence of other people, fear of filling out receipts, checks or any other documents in the presence of third parties) are less common.

How does sociophobia relate?

Maintenance rates are generally calculated by the amount of time you spend and the amount of money you spend. Admittedly, this is a very popular song that has been around for some time. Many people enjoy a great deal of fun, even if they have no choice but to share it with others. Obviously this is the most important situation in the situation. According to sociophobics, the current situation is normalized by the process of gaining a foothold. If you do not want to miss the opportunity, the sociophobia will take advantage of the form. Clearly, on the other hand, it is possible to unravel, especially, if there is a traditional Secrets of Social phobia in this area.

We've a primer. Mister B. should be clearly separated from the same data. It is a common school of thought and in the world of women. There are no psychological problems that can not be exploited by anyone (even if they do not work). The result is that the steel does not have any problems with other people and it is not possible to find a way out. I have a very strange subject, which can not be freely shared with people. Buttons, which are considered to be the most expensive. Explain the value of all items that you have, and that you will not find out what you are doing in this category.

What does sociophobia mean?

The sociophobia of education can be explained to people, such as women and women, by the way they are taught and the way they are treated. For example, homeownership can be shared by those who are not affiliated with any other branch, such as one.

28

notify you about the performance of the problem with the user, and the user can change the distance between each user.

How does sociophobia work?

The origins of sociophobia for self-esteem are declining. However, sociophobia describes a psychotropic situation, it is malignant. Explain different predictions. One of them is something that the rebbe imitates sociophobically. Another is to limit the development of social skills: if a person does not know how to behave in a particular situation, then this can cause anxiety and excitement. The role of the game is not played or the number of characters on the list is not calculated. It is well known that the predisposition to the past tense can also be maintained.

What are the sociophobic issues?

Conversations show that people with sociophobia are more likely to have no choice but to change their minds. In addition, they often have problems getting an education, as fear of the group and public speaking can greatly interfere with the learning process, even to the point of its termination. In such cases, as the case may be, there are serious differences in the current rate. If you want to get rid of alcohol, many people will give you alcohol, which you take for granted.

Episodes of depression are also characteristic of the people, the traditional sociophobia.

2.3. Sociology phobias

Research shows that the most effective way to treat this problem is through medical treatment and over-the-counter therapy.

29

Medical commentary

The most popular are the antidepressants (antidepressants). The distinguished class of antidepressants is known as the MAIO, nprimimer, and maclobemid inhibitors. They are effective on Secrets of Social phobias, in chastity, on social media. Physical sympathetic symptoms can be seen in the results of beta-blockers (propranolol or atenolol). It is specified in the most recent search terms that are used by physics, such as printers, printers, and printers. Sessional measures of the most effective effect of the first-degree antidote that any drug contains. In the most common three-dimensional treatment, the medical treatment of adverse therapies is not limited to.

Custody therapy

Corrosive orienteering therapies for steady-state reduction of symptoms. At the same time, the therapeutic work of the non-partisans will be divided, which will be the first of all symptoms and which will be addressed. The assertion is supported in the subdivision plan. An expert in specialist therapy provides methods and techniques, the effectiveness of which is applied to the work that we are doing. In the process of using trapezoidal patients, the full range of properties, such as size, size, size.

In the following therapies, sociophobics are divided into three groups:

1. The working number of the working tree.
2. Writing social scores.

Provision of assessments.

There are three ways to combine, as well as to use a different type of drug.

30

Working t-shirt design works

It is also known as cognitive therapy (definition = mycelium). The first step is to track negative thoughts (e.g., "I'm sure I'm going to get shivering," or "They'll think I'm a nerd," or "It's going to be terrible if he doesn't like me").

Tailor-made models for the day, which are shared by the most important part of the team. The possibilities of transformation are even more realistic and steady.

Establishment of social news

Indeed, in the most biased sociophobic tribe, the most common is the socialist nobility. The risk of not responding to anything that the person can do is not visible at the time of presentation to the user. The acquisition of social skills usually occurs in a group setting, where in the process of role-playing games, certain social situations are simulated, discussed and played out.

Addition of attachments

Pre-therapy can not be done specifically, because it is not pre-emptive. Very effective "on-screen" promotion, based on situational, provocative travel. We are particularly fond of simple situations, especially with them. Patients, copyers, can write to the store, store in the store the broken item or you have a copy of it. Trivia, which is used to fulfill ethical challenges, will definitely be appreciated. When performing such tasks, a person discovers that the negative effect he expects is not true, and he approaches the next situation with a great sense of self-confidence.

31

We will use the key elements of real-time therapy and the phobia of solving problems. It cuts physical pressure and obliges the completion of other drills.

The moment of fulfillment of each of the following polynomial therapies will be recognized by the patient. If you are interested in the "Work in progress" category, please refer to it and follow the reviews. We maintain an overview, which is based on the evaluation of negative moments. This can be used in periodic tableware and day-to-day debugging. One of the most important results of the results is that this is a product.

The logo, the patient prefixed the frame, the frame in the first frame shows the width and width. There is a lot of power and energy involved. We do not have a lot of energy and we have to deal with a lot of problems, we have a lot of people with nothing. Many people, analyzing their processes, try to outline the prevalence of sociophobia. One design works that energizes and enables one to succeed in completing practical exercises. Obviously, in the case of protracted lesions, there is a difference in the size of the patient, the specific type of lesion.

If you find this information helpful, please try 3.

2.4. Suggest your next level

If you want to get rid of clutter, update your troubleshooting issues. In addition to the number of messages sent by multiple users, we recommend that you re-select your name.

For this full test (scales of Leiboviza), the value of your level of activity and stress in a different social class.

Forward to "Work Themes" and complete Exercise 4.

32

Be brave in your own special level. You will be prompted to return to this test. This allows you to evaluate the effect of the workflow.

You will be able to take advantage of one or the other test, which will distinguish your personal equipment. If you are looking for "Test situation", you can also find it in "Work topics".

Forward to "Work Themes" and complete Exercise 5.

You will be able to use your level on the "Test situation" - this is a test case that you will find in the building.

2.5. Prepayment of your sociophobia

If you are logged in as part of 2.3, you will find three types of sociophobia. In practical work with social situations, you can also use the post workout. Pre-streamlining results in a convenient situation where you have the same control over your trip. This is the most effective way to solve a problem. In category 6 plays, you can create a plan for the successful delivery of HeleMogo.

It is not yet time to start a breeze on your trip, as you

will be able to log in and select a "good" game. This will increase your chances of winning.

In some cases, you may need to upgrade your mobile network to find out what the problem is.

You will find some trivia that you can use to differentiate yourself from the most rational issues. This is what makes the most successful result in this situation. When selecting and remembering your mouse, you will find it in level 3.

Let's help you find what you are looking for. This is discussed in Chapter 4. As soon as you learn how to do this, then with a little practice you can quickly reach a state of relaxation, which will be useful when performing subsequent exercises.

3 - 2756

33

The other types of items listed below are listed in heading 5. You will need to check the range if this is the case. We're cracking it, it's sliding down and down the razor blade. I was immediately approached by a very difficult situation, especially if I was correctly referring to something in the process.

In this case, the predominant means of completing propositions, which may be of different denominations, may be different. First of all, the solution to the problem is that the main theme is the same theme. Poetry can be used as a relaxation exercise, all of which work on the third floor. Shape the tag, which you can perform on a flat screen, or work with a quarter. We definitely recommend them: one of the three glasses, which is usually used to complete the design.

Provider handling deletes sufficient amounts of time. Do not overdo it. Remember that the time required to complete the application is to increase the number of applications.

These are the ones that can be used to work on your own issues.

3. Determining Negative Miscellaneous

3.1. Emotion of emotion

Present what you want to read in the past and the list of issues in the community. What are you talking about? Clearly, silently spit out. There is no sign yet. For example, if you are looking for a vase, you should try to find out what you are looking for in the picture.

The program does not automatically state the last one. Let me know what I think about the subject, and let me know what I mean. You are not logged in. In the description of the various scenarios, we sent automated and millennial dummies to grabbers, assembled at home. This is the state of the art, which is a wonderful place to meet people.

This is a schematic diagram which shows:

1) society,

2) thought,

3) power.

This is a primer.

You're getting stretched out with the drug. It is recommended that you pay attention to what you are doing, and that you do not know how to do it. How are you doing? The most important things you can expect are different: the size, the size, the size of the box, the size of the part and the color of each part. d. Everything you see is what you think of it. Note: "It will always be punctual. Clearly, what was going on. It is possible to have a different one ». That which is in vain, and that which is in vain, and that which is in vain, and that which is in vain, is that which is in vain.

I'm for no one does not know."

35

It is possible to wash your hand and remove your debris at this point in time.

3.2. Development of companies, municipalities and companies

Delete this is not always easy. Submit search results (this is the first or last call). This is an objective fact.

Note: "Customers will be able to select the item and the folder to open", "My message will save my item". You can test, test and save as much as you can, as a fixed fix and video.

The size of the window, the size of the "I view, which I do not understand", is the newest possible feature of the video camera. You can see if there is another window in the window, you will see a quote. You can set the default or unbound path to the path you are interested in. However, such an exclusion does not make it any more objective, it is just a matter of time. There are some things that you can do to get rid of them, but you can tell them what they are and what they are.

Muesli, outstanding subjects, which we do not associate with. The "My source will" message will be your interpreter. In this case, the part of the item is the subject of the "predicted note in them" or, possibly, "serial version".

The words "They do not work for me" and "I do not love you" are just a few words, but this one is not a new one. Taki mice do not have a logical output of faults. The tool interprets the most important facts about the most recent version. If a person has a quarrel with them that he or she is in, then he or she does not know what he or she is. If you are in such a situation, you will be using the same topic, which will be edited in the same way as anyone else.

36

It's not possible to delete messages from memory.

The words "I remember, what you do not know", "I remember, what you want to do" will work again. There are only two types of windows and three windows that can be used for different types of windows.

In the table, 1 level indicates the number of values, and then - the number of cases, the number of cases in the case.

Table 1 August and medial processes

Lust	Mysli
Pechal	Potato cocoa or cheek libo; unite all units
Power	It's obnoxious or it's all that goes into your cell
Development	Finding something that is not nice
The city	Contact or contact us

It is very important to understand and distinguish between objects, objects and places. This is a problem that can be effectively remedied in problematic situations.

Release with Exercise Exercise 6.

3.3. Periodical analysis of mycelium

In this case, the size of the part, as well as the size, size and size of the part of the item. In fact, this is what we analyze in our analysis. User analysis of the most

common news item:
DATE
2. SUBJECT
3. USTVO
4. MUSIC
37
You will find all that you have selected and all of them are selected. This is the analysis of the microscope analysis. The distribution of goods and services generally does not represent a value; selection This feature has many nice features.
Note: "The document will not be sent to the city". It is important to remember that you are a company and a company. Occupation (physiological leveling) is the subject, and time - the subject. It is possible for you to make a donation, as long as you have a share in the sale of your property.
Let us first analyze the microscope: "One thinks that what we have not done. It's good, I'm shooting an idiot ».
DATE: August 16
ASSEMBLY: This is what you find most beautiful and beautiful.
FASHION: trip, city.
MUSIC: it feels like nothing is happening to it, it's good, something's idiotic.
This is the prime minister: "I love you very much." O should be highlighted with Victor and superimposed on it. He, on the other hand, has always been a fan. It will be very easy to remember ». For those who have successfully completed the "Work in progress", it is necessary to follow the following instructions:
DATE: May 13th.
SUBJECT: Get rid of links with Victor. TASK: travel, city.

MUSIC: it is a well-built, well-maintained unit that can hold up to a month.
Successfully complete the challenge 7.
You can save your trip from missiles to existing items. In this case, there are a number of difficult problems that can be solved and provoked through the process. We recommend that you make sure you follow the instructions below. In the
38
this new moment is not a sovereign deity, but every missile.
In the case of a random analysis, you can specify the following values:
DATE: 12 December.
ASSEMBLY: This is a cross domaine.
FUTURE: wellness, travel.
MUSIC: I do not have the right to exit.
One of these analyzes analyzes one of the most common problems, which is what is involved in nerves. In this case, the analysis is successful: when you react, you are in the middle of a series of missiles and chambers that you have. The description of the SABETIs applications is based on the specificity of the SABTISTI system of the three micelles. Note also:
DATE: 12 December.
ASSEMBLY: extension (duma om nem).
FUTURE: Trivia.
MUSIC: it's something that you'll be able to forge.
If you are interested in a topic that you are looking for, enter the previous entry in the "SUBJECT" graph. If you want, you can add "duma a ...", but it is not obvious.
A series of prequels to complete quests 8.
3.4. Analyze your books and pictures
The same analysis is performed on you, which you will

find on the same page, the number and the number of them. You can get the most out of it in a very specific way in your "Work Tops" section, which is clearly defined.

39

Remember, you're taking a break. You specify, what kind (when you remember) you have the same name (name, number of characters). As you can see, what happened to you during the period when you are going to get acquainted and enjoy yourself. Note: "It is possible, however, that we do not know what is good for you".

If you just want to save something on a daily basis:

DATE: July 1st.

ASSEMBLY: meeting the needs of our dealers. TASK: trivia, appraisal.

MUSIC: they are the ones that are not good enough for you.

Release with Exercise Exercise 9.

When you execute the "Work topic", you will be prompted to enter a position.

On average, we do not specify the intensity of your treatment. For this scale, scales range from 0 to 100 bales. 100 Balls are selected by different characters, each of which can be used to select 0 balloons. If you want to get rid of it, you should try to get rid of it, as it is not possible to sell it at 50 or so.

These vehicles, which are distributed, are provided in a convenient and up-to-date manner by the municipality. The number of cases that need to be specified in the percentage is true (the number of participants). 100% deserves absolute approval, 0% - full failure of your predicament.

Well, the people in the prime of the world can

appreciate what you have done to each other, the ones that need to be different. In the case of sludge, it is possible to post a 10% follow-up to that muesli.
Please note that the following changes are made:
DATE: July 1st.
ASSEMBLY: the distance of the taps.
40
FUTURE: trip, registration (50). MUSEUM: I do not have a single good news for you (10%).
Listed in the form below, in which case the form, if any, shall not be included. You need to be aware of what you are looking for, as long as it is available on your own. When it comes to the distribution of your devices, you will not find the current problem, the problem is different.
It is also necessary to use affirmative forms of your thoughts instead of the intended ones: that is, not "Maybe they will think that I am a little strange," but "They will think that I am strange." The description of such words, such as "can be" and "enough", you can change the number of percentages of a sentence. Note: "They think they are foreign (25%)". Even if you do, you will not be able to reach the top of your page. You will be exposed to the percentages of your missiles.
Prevent Execution 10.
The "Working Themes" event enables you to select the most important objects. We, in the first instance, have decided that we should close the exam on the part of the auditor.
DATE: 13 December.
ASSEMBLY: Examination of the auditorial test (duma om etom).
FASHION: Trivia, Panika (80).

MUSIC: it can be very nerve-wracking, as it is not possible to remove the sample from the liver (20%). I did not take the exam (25%). We have a very small amount of dowry (10%).

It is important to evaluate the size, size and size of the crop and the intensity of the growth. The most important part of the journey, it is said, is that there are some missiles, but the intensity is 80

41

Balls are very clear. What can be said is that it contains many other things, which are not the same.

Note: "If you do not have an exam, you will not need it either" or "If you do not know what you are doing." Takiy Mysli provides 80 percent of the rides. The poem was once called the "Working Thread" event. Suggest new wood-based paint jobs that are not straightforward. You can easily find the following:

1) a certain number, a prime minister, such as: «What can I project? What is it? What does this mean? ”; " What is the best way to project?", "What is unique about each one?";

2) used, which can be used. This is the technology we use to describe "Promote cinema cinema". The bolshnevta lüdee tend tend to have a cocoa-liba simanoialis, which is completely unmistakable. One of these is why you tend to have these tendencies, or you have to take advantage of this method. In addition, any negative data that can be concretized and distributed will be displayed on the screen. It is safe to assume that you will be able to select the desired size.

All you have to do is fill out all the instructions, such as the size of the project. Definitely worthwhile, you can analyze, what you want and what you have to do with it. First page, all prompting and trying to find the

following position:
1. Project management - is it something concrete and objective or just a mix of things, money, ideas or things? What does it look like when it comes to fixing video cameras?
2. Is there a problem with the number of bases, branches, as well as the wind, wine, city, snow, rainfall, rain or snow? Can this be
42
hidden under the mist of the mistletoe, the prime minister, "Oh, the goddess, who did not love him"?
3. Did the missile manifestation or the missile inversion occur? Are they in the form of an extractor?
4. Do you miss your books, what do you think is the intent of the books? If not, then the purpose is to create a unique mix, which is the purpose of the promotion.

You can configure how to completely remove your messenger.

Exercises 11, 12, 13.

3.5. Continuous analysis of mycelium

These are the types of equipment that can be used to analyze your mice and animals, such as the "Warehouse" section. Each day, in addition to that moment, you will be dealing with such a workaround. You will be able to concentrate on your subjects and children, which will make you sociophobic. Generally, when driving or traveling. You list in the "Working topic" that you are the one, the most intense and intense. Let's tell you, what kind of relationship do you have or what do you think you do? The next item is the same item. You will need to remember which cookies were used by you. You will find and report as many different things as possible, even if you do not know what they are and what they are. Challenge yourself, as you can see the professionalism of the more sophisticated premium technology.

One thing is for sure, we have all the files in one of the applications. There is no page on this page. The actual car parts, which are supposedly decorated in different colors.

If you want to create a new page, you can specify the number of pages that you want to display.

43

The "They think they are stupid" mouse does not have the same theme as the "They think it is stupid" thing. "It's not enough to save me," it says, "But it's something I've been missing for a while."

There are many types of custom-built windows that can be used to move, adjust or disassemble. These exercises will help you to avoid negative thoughts and feelings about what you are not doing in the control room. This is unnecessary. It is not uncommon for you to find out what you are doing, which will help you to understand what is going on. For this purpose, the vehicle will be able to view and distribute negative missiles.

Complete the task 14.

3.6. Rational and irrational missiles

Misli is a product that is constantly being updated with the same content. We'll just swear and kill you. The mail you are about to retrieve, which is not a bad thing at all. If you delete another file, save it with the specified name, if the code is set to 3.1, do not specify an error. If you are a fan of fanaticism, you will find that this is a very nice place to live. We work with a lot of people who deal with specific developments in the process.

Irrational mice - these are mice, which are not clearly fitted. They do not provide real facts. Note, for example, "All things you can do when you send your notebook". It is often assumed that nothing from this item is being stored. Or you say: "I do not know who I am, I do not know what to do", which is the only part of the application to send.

Rational mice - these are real mice. They logically extract from real subjects. If you are in a state of despair, you will be deprived of your support, you will be saved, and you will be rewarded with what you know.

available »provides a rational rationale. If the hostess of the party approaches you with an outstretched hand when you enter the room, it is also rational to assume that she wants to shake your hand and greet you. Rational missiles do not always have positive

results. If it's what you're criticizing, it's natural that it's predisposed to what you've been up to at the moment. One such irrational dummy that this guy is pissed off about. These are the ones that have been criticized by some as a result of this - this is what the rationalists say.
As a result, the emphasis is on the logical logistics, primer, and secondary processing. This is what the key is to provide an open source of information on different types of links. Note: "You do not have a lot of fun", "They are not very good at anything", neither are they.
The second primer will be displayed in the "select hidden fields" field. This means that a person pays much more attention to negative events, even greatly exaggerates them, while the positive aspects of the event remain behind the scenes. For example, a key that exits in presentations, which is not a single product: «It has not been updated. I do not think so. Practically no issues. One of the slides occupies the pervert ». This article does not cover positive facts, which are considered to be relevant to this topic.
3.7. Missile meaning
If you have a different level of performance in your game, you will find that it is possible to create a new one in the new one. This moment adds a four-dimensional shape, which is called the "microscope shape". Butterflies that can be dispensed with can be used to irradiate irradiated lice and to reduce lumps of dehydration.
45
Suggestions for basic memory settings:
• Tactical development (section 3.7);
• new opiate, the position of the non-volatility of your

muesli (ratio 3.8).
Determine, distribute, and wash your hands rationally and keep them real. This can be done by trying to sort out standard wizards. Define the current accounts for each month, which you will find in the hotel.
This is what makes the most successful BREAKTHROUGH PERFORMANCE PERSONALITY OF SWEDISH MUSEUM.
By default you will be able to access all types of files that can be used for all applications.
1. Do you want to save your money on a regular basis, if you have a problem with it?
2. How, by my knowledge, do other things happen to you in the most favorable situations?
3. Can I hear something on the radio, or see it on TV, or read it in a book or magazine, or learn from other people that would prove the veracity of my thought?
4. Can this nibble do not cover the possible effects?
5. Can the other people (can we name it specifically) do you think so, who and what?
6. If this is the case with a lot of people: "Make sure you think about it, if the situation is different"!
7. Are there any other reasons why you and your family are interested in what specific facts can be explained?
8. Can I have the same situations with other types of media that can be used? If so, what is the status of the company? (You will be logged in to the NOW MUSEUM graph).

46

There are several types of applications and variants that you can use to specify the level of rationality of your choice. If you have any issues or issues, please contact us. In fact, you can use irrational mosquitoes,

which can be punished, but not in the corn. Poetry you are the new mice, the most common.
Note:
DATE: April 17th.
TOTAL: Submit a message to my friend.
FUTURE: Wall (80).
MUSIC:
1. I have water-water power (95).
2. One thinks that what is an idiot is true (80). MUSIC WORK:
1. It is beautiful, but it does not have a rough shape, which is a dome on it.
I do not want to send the message to another user.
2. It is important to note that these products are not and will not be stored,
what you have not been able to verify, this is an idiot. The news item is very good at T., and all of it is crisp.
NEW MUSIC:
1. Well, this is the ability to do what is right, but it's not a good idea, but it's a great one.
2. If you want to get rid of it, it's not going to work, but it's going to waste. Possibly, for this one will not be able to make any concessions.
You can configure what works in the database and you can create the most common one in the "Workplace" section, which is used interchangeably. Do not overwrite most of them. This is the moment when you will be participating in the "Work in progress" section. Can be used for practical work with our mice, and the color is available for all types of delays. This will not allow you to override your prediction with other tools.
47
and zrenia. If you choose to use this tool, you will see a similar effect.

You can use the best information about the logical logs in the selected sociophobics and what you can do with them

You can also try to find a solution in the form of a sample, preferably by size. 42-43.

3.8. Candidate experiments

One example of this is the analysis of the microscope:

This set of irrational microscopic values is based on the new output, which indicates the desired value. You can test tests for information about the variability of your mice (or there are outbreaks). This is a very special experiment.

You can send another message: «What do you want to save? These are the ones that were left by T. how are you What do you think about ...? » And so on.

On the other hand, it is possible to select the name of the item, the reaction of the people to your mailbox, which will try to save your item. For example, if you think people will make sarcastic remarks to you if you leave the party first, then the best way to check it out is to leave the party early one day. If all else fails, it's the same thing you can do to try it out. Predominantly treacherous prediction of an unreliable repository. In the example above, they'll presumably make the following remark, "Did your mommy set a curfew for you?", Or "Are you on a leash?" or something like that.

48

This is a prime example: a person who thinks that no one will not be able to take a vow will not be able to reach them. On the other hand, it seems that many other things do not attract the attention of people with disabilities. A possible behavioral experiment would be as follows: do not start any conversations and conversations at the party (just stand and look around) and observe whether they really do not start talking to him.

Experiment with what you need to know about your topic, which really works. If your predispositions are negligible, you will end up experimenting, you will be able to get rid of them irrationally.

Thus, after each analysis of thoughts, you talk about the possibility of setting up a behavioral experiment that will provide you with information about the reliability of your assumptions.

In the first part of the program, the number of characters specified in paragraph 3.7 shall be different from the number one character. It's a logo, it's possible to spread the word, it's a one-size-fits-all suit, and it's a one-size-fits-all one. The most common phobia that can be used to successfully complete the kaki-libo experiment. If there are any issues with this topic, please note that each one, if any, is the same as this one.

Complete the task 15.

3.9. Logical errors
and irrational mice,
the most repulsive of sociophobia

However, it is very important that you analyze all of your musculoskeletal disorders. It is my intention to observe logical teachings, especially the emphasis on sociophobia. You can include predisposed primary and secondary experiments in your previous analysis.

4—2756

49

This is a sociophobic tradition, in particular, distinguishes one from another, one that does not differ from one another. You can try to find out which features are right for you.

1. You will find specific / relevant information (smell, appearance, ignition of your appearance) as you will see.
2. As you know, no specific information is used to determine the value of other products.
3. As you know, many other things are mentioned in your message.
4. As you can see, what you are looking for is a good way to get rid of clutter you don't need.
5. You think that what you are talking about is a bad memory of what you are doing or what is happening to you.

Exercises 16 and 17.

Logical error № 1:

The true nature of the concrete realization

The people of the city, the traditional sociophobia, do not need to know what they are / what they are about. It is possible that if you do not have one, you can change the following:

• the smell of smoke, enough or cold;
• unobtrusive advertising;
• closure;
• throw in the glass;
• shared photo sharing;
• unpaved pages;
• Custom debit or custom debugging.

It is also possible to create real estate, and some of the most important things to do are to enjoy a unique experience. What is happening, what is happening, what is happening?

50

there are many things that we owe to you. Copy, paste, print, paste, paste, paste, paste, paste, paste, tap, tap, tap, tap, tap.

Poetry can be differentiated, it is possible to predict the prediction of that or any other physical phenomenon. If you think that you have been exposed to all sorts of issues on your own, that's what's a new topic ', please see:

• When analyzing your thoughts, make sure that you are really afraid of the appearance of the signs described above (for example, "my hands will tremble", "I will not be able to say a word", "sweat will drain from my forehead").

• Analyze if there is a problem, distribute it, and do not use it as a means of restraint, with the help of solutions, preferably in the 3rd grade.

Complete the task 18.

Provide relevant experiments with tachymlysms. Check out the "Working topics" section.

Complete the task 19.

Logical error № 2:

The truth of the matter is that the other party will change your mind

Another possible logical fallacy is that some of your physiological phenomena or appearance traits (e.g., being overweight, having a big nose) will necessarily be noticed by other people. This is a socio-phobic tradition that tends to negatively interpret the reaction of others. It is possible that you will not be able to get any information about this item, but that it will be the same as the one you have.

At the same time, there are many other people who can name a lot of them. From here, things get trickier, and this is where the true love comes from!

51

positive aspects of self-promotion with scribes. You will not be able to find out what you are looking for in the box. It is considered to be the most important source of information, as it is not known to anyone. Suppose, first, or at least one of them is ready for you. If all that you are looking for, characterize and for your situation, according to the "Working topics" category:

• Be aware of the fact that you have been given similar data by analyzing your mouse. Note: "If you want to play, X. I'm going to hide", "If you want to get rid of it, I'm going to get rid of it".

• Analyze if there are any problems, as well as if they are related to each other, as well as the number of cases in which there are three.

Complete the task 20.

Provide possible experimental experiments with mycelium video. Meet in "Workplaces", as it were.

Execution events 21, 22, 23 and 24.

Logical Exhibit № 3: The value of this, which is another form of negative reminiscence of your remembrance, the remembrance

The tradition of the sociophobics is that we believe that we do not know how to make a lot of money. They can easily be displayed in glasses or other slips, which for this purpose are not unusual. I have no choice but to drop out of another glass vase type "Wow, what a wow!" or you will find out that all the vouchers are closed. Predisposition, which is the second most pronounced in the negative part, is called the "middle name". If you are not

you are telephoning, this is the one you need to write a review about. It is said that the traditional sociophobic "quote" is one of the most important ones in this one. The reactions of other people are not exactly the same as the prediction of the most

important ones.
What is the nature, the nature, the nature and the nature of the subject, are not even those that are (and are not). Other people in the classroom are open to the public, as well as sociophobics, as many as we can.
If you have any issues, please refer to your site, if you want to follow the topic «Working topics»:
• In the process of analyzing the various types of products that have been used, we have been able to identify different types of type. Note: "If you want to delete the item you are looking for, you can select the one you want to use."
• Analyze if there are any problems, as well as if they are not related to the development of data, which can be used in the process of recovery.
Complete the challenge 25
Delete possible data experiments with your mouse video. Check out the "Working topics" section.
Complete the task 26.
Logical error № 4: The ability of the tag that does not appear to be similar to that of the "associated" scale
All of them are located in the situation, which is the type of variance that your "destination" will have on one or the other
53
we play, which can be negatively related to each other. Tradition sociopophobia that deletes logical logos, the number of which is a predetermined value, which is one of them. Even if you do not, you will be exposed to the negative aspects of your cellularity. One thing that happens is that the other people do not have access to any of the "items" in any of them. Traditional sociophobia is concentrated on the negative aspects of self-promotion as well as this one.

If, for some reason, you are interested in your situation, please follow the steps below.

• Analyze your mouse, make sure what you are trying to get your mouse to type. For example: "If they notice my stiffness, they will think that I am a churban", "If they look at me with a grin when my hands tremble, they will think that I am a complete neurotic."

• Analyze if there are any problems, as well as if they are not related to the development of data, which can be used in the process of recovery.

ATTENTION!

Analyze your mouse, do you want to know what you think you are about to do? It is possible, in the character of a person, that you are going to be married, these are typical neurotic cards. What do you think other people can do to save money on what, if anything, at all? It is possible that you are a socialist.

Complete the task 27.

•Delete possible data experiments with your mouse video. Meet in "Workplaces", as it were.

54

Exercises 28 and 29.

Lots of people, traditional sociophobia, shit, what is a good thing and nothing to do with it and what we do. We have specified this as a clone in connection. For example, a person who has been criticized for several typing errors may think that other people think they are completely unfit for the job. Otherwise it can shoot, which even the popularity of this one, after all, and the anecdotes. Anything that is unique to one another may not work properly. There is no doubt about it, and it is clear from this that we have not been able to find a way out yet. If you are looking for something else that is completely different from the other negative aspect of it (please note) this is a very successful post. There are many other things that can be discussed in this article, including the good, the bad, the intelligent, and the ones we have. d.

If you want to use one of these tools, you will be able to use the various options. The unidirectional thinking of a person suffering from Secrets of Social phobia contributes to the fact that he begins to idealize others for no particular reason, relying only on one of their positive aspects. Taking advantage of the misconceptions that we may have in the alternative are possible.

Complete the task 30.

Another person, a traditional sociophobia, says: It's because it's expensive, it's on the phone, it's a real predicament for the sake of it.

If you want to get rid of clutter, you can use the following password:

55

Logical error № 4:

Predominance of items that are covered by each item from your favorite products or products

Let's try a different experiment, which summarizes the prediction of logical objects.

Make sure you keep track of the company, up to 100 people. Well, when it comes to housing, it's a prime minister (especially, you'll be proud of it). You will find that there is a large number of people you are referring to (point 1).

If this is a project, it will be calculated, then, 20 points out of 100 (point 2).

Of those, 20 are not rated as negative, and, I think, a few - 10 points (point 3).

Out of 10 10 each, 20% of each item is similar to

another item (item 4).
It's worth mentioning that in groups of 100 people need only two, which are separated from each other by the number of trials. It is not possible for a person to shoot a bullet that has a positive impact on it, but even if it does. Destroy some objects, but do not use them in this case. Release the key (!) Which does not work.
As you can see, the number of negative reactions can be different from the ones you have selected. Anyway, it's possible, you need two locks from each cover, which are connected to each other negatively. This is a sociophobic tradition, which preserves the meaning of the logical phrase: they are the ones that are different from one another. It is not uncommon for them to have a bad nightmare and not be able to reach a certain level.
Nectar does not have any concrete reactions from the pots. We have the same size as the ones that are "folded" in the glass, not filled with any of the custom windows. For example, "I'm sorry to hear that", "I have all the criticisms".
56
If you have any special requirements or situations, you can use the following instructions for the "Work" section:
• Analyze your mouse, make sure that you do not accidentally touch your mouse to a specific type. For example: "If they don't like me, they will never come to visit me again," "They think I'm too nervous and they'll tell everyone," "If he thinks I'm worthless, then I'm really worthless."
• Analyze if there are any problems, as well as if they are not related to the development of data, which can

be used in the process of recovery.
If you think that the consequences of rejection of you by other people will be expressed mainly in a cold attitude towards you, then these questions are a good way to check whether your thoughts correspond to reality.
There are many other types of pages that you can create from there, which are not the most unique ones you have. Note: "I want to share", "I want to share", "I do not want to criticize you". In the case of a successful call to your predecessor, it will not be up-to-date. Can you save the same number: can I try not to use the same version?
In the process of resolving your issue, please contact:
"If you need to find someone, you will not be logged in." If you find yourself in a situation where it's not a bad thing. It is common to have a company of 100 people: a couple, a couple of people, a couple of people, it is not possible to work with them.
This is a good idea - keep an eye on the best. If you have any issues with this topic, please do not hesitate to contact us. If you want to respond to negative feedback about yourself, then what they are doing will not be read to you. Well, if you're going to have to lie down and talk to someone who's talking about it, that's all you do.
57
money or anything. If it is you who are stupid, needy and selfish, and you are, they are not, and they are what they are.
If you react to the negative judgment of others because you agree with them, then you should work through this agreement: how you have come to this belief over the years, to such low self-esteem. It's

sledding away is something like a pomegranate or a psychotherapist.

Complete the task 31.

•Delete possible data experiments with your mouse video. Meet in "Workplaces", as it were.

Exercises 32 and 33.

We observe that we are all logical logos, which are dominated by people, traditional sociophobia.

When you fill in the "Thoughts" column in your daily report at the end of the day, you need to stop and ask yourself if you have made one or more of the logical errors described above. You need to try to get rid of all your problems in the most difficult logical way possible.

3.10. Other challenges
by irrational missile design

1. It is with the sociophobia that forms a negative image. The negative and irrational mix of what you are talking about is what you are talking about. For this purpose, you must specify that the world and each other have the same name. For this you can na-

that is the PREVIOUS DENVICES vest, which can be used to indicate your positive views and views. Make sure you have no rating or value, do not specify the value of each key, whether "or" or not. Recall that you have checked your receipts. These can be used to save large amounts of time for the maintenance of such services. Some may find that they seem to have a very good understanding of what is going on. This is an example of a day when you want to share all the compliments.

Please note that at the end of a positive day you will not be able to find any recent records:

• list unsecured claims;
• evaluate or delete private views;
• Include all additional features.

Complete the task 34.

*2.*We have a lot of heroes, that people, a traditional sociophobia, a scumbag, that is going to be negatively charged with nothing. If you have a slippery slope and are slightly overgrown with it, you will see a good amount of it in the middle of nowhere. Bolshevism of the bastard is a critique of what we are talking about. In situations where the emotions are constantly evolving, the traditional sociophobia is related to what it is all about. The whole thing looks like a strange thing that you're proud of. This is a very nice product, as it's not a good one at all. This does not mean that it is possible to occupy the upper part of the vehicle. If you want to be able to use the display, you can easily select the one you want to use.

Complete the task 35.

3. Possessing the unproductive practices of a positive movement, the use of such practices, as well as

59

You can formulate a positive setting. For example, "I can have a dowry; I have a lot of good news ». Even the plants do not have the ability to express phrases. All of your key features are defined in previous events. Admittedly, it's a constant source of confusion that you can not even boast of a positive attitude.

Complete the task 36.

4. NEW BENEFITS

4.1. Login

In addition, the maintenance of the tires on the vehicle is free of charge, which does not cause any damage to it or not. In this case, you will need to make the necessary recommendations, as well as the specifics, which you will be able to follow.

4.2. Unknown message

There is no such thing as what you are going to do, and what you are going to do. You can use the "good, not bad" design to create a warm, upholstered look. If you want to get rid of it, it's a great idea to add a glass to the glass that you are looking for.

Also, the time at which the data is displayed will be displayed on the screen.

Contact Glazes

Look at other parts, which you can choose from, and the size of the straps will be covered with only the glass, which will be a product. Which ones do you prefer?

Leap of air

Exercising your weight is a great way to enhance your lifestyle. The poem is not valid, which can be separated by the one you want to delete.

61

Telephony

Get rid of clutter you need, keep your cooler and cooler. Do not slow down, save or stop forwarding. Do not wash your clothes and clothes, they will not work.

Range of manure

Remember that you need to be able to grumble and play (not tartarit). Light and not monotonous.

Some of the most recent reports have been published by new publishers. The poet will complete the

practical exercises.
Exercises 43 - 49.

4.3. Start a task

The file does not appear to be real. To this end, as the first word is displayed, it is necessary to have a constant non-verbal contact. You will find in version 4.2 that you will be able to access glaze contact. It is easy to get rid of clutter you don't need, as long as you keep it cool. The number of applications, which are clearly related to specific and specific applications - is one that is referred to as "translation".

Note:

- Solid / Curvy / Pleasant shade.
- Do you need enough time?
- Try to secure.
- What is your favorite?
- How much did you spend?
- This is a slippery slope.
- Which cohort did you find?
- Etc.

62

The size of the ball bearing, which is the case with the bracket shown in the frame, is the value of each part. If you have already started a conversation with someone, you can change the topic of conversation, so you will create comfortable conditions for your interlocutor, who may be embarrassed by your "invasion". Bad slick slides do not work well.

Complete the challenge 50.

4.4. Support message: list of users

Lots of people are talking about what they are going to do in a moment of need. If you want to get out of here, you should be able to do whatever you want, as long as you have no interest in the subject. You can send the name of the name to the name you want to create. Many people find the most important thing in the blogger's list.

Indeed, what you have not learned, what you have done. Here are some suggestions on how to look or get an appointment for antique items. You can delete this, complete the process and demonstrate it with the best interest (do not change it).

Descending and sacred proclamations

Declared vouchers - these vouchers, which are called "what", "what", "where", "who", "how" and so on. d.

Note: And what do you think is this one?

- What are you developing?
- Who are you dating?

Secret vouchers - these vouchers, on which you can vote only "to" or "not". Note:

- What do you think is this?

63

- Who likes to work on a roof?
- Do you work in the office?

Butterflies do not represent the power of the hurricane, which is what the hurricane is about. Incredible names are very useful for supporting communities. Shelter, which regularly adjusts the output, which is used to display the value of the item.

Exercises 51, 52 and 53.

Subject of thematic issues

Get rid of clutter you can pry on one and the same theme. For example, if it's a culinary business, it's possible to swear by a lot of bloodshed or restaurant and barristers. You will be presiding over certain topics, which will be covered by your subordinate. Do not disconnect from the theme on the theme, rather secure one line in the frame. So, if you continue to talk about foreign cuisine, you can ask how your interlocutor liked certain dishes, how often he was abroad, what he thinks about it, etc. You are not allowed to listen to anything and you are only required to do so. Time from time to time may be delegated to the owner or to the recipients. It does not always have data, which is the source of the message. If you want to get started, you can easily share your badges, even if you do,

Other types of support cases

Remember that you can save messages and other messages. If you are interested in the "Mmmmm ..." prediction, you should check your interest, not the first submission. When the government takes a break, you can stay

64

neskolko slov, naprimerir, «Desteistvitelne? d. Another thing you can easily post is the following word for your subject: "Great three things!"

One of the most effective methods used is the scaling method. Note: "Yes, it's all there is to it, what you are talking about."

Complete exercises 54 and 55.

4.5. Heaviness protection

The power supply is not capable of securing the power of the other power supply. Also, as for the most important part of this, for the purpose of maintaining the most consistent and clear phrases:

- Nice to meet you. Take a look at Jonah.
- This is of particular interest, but it is not a wealth of gold / gold. It will take a while to recover.
- It's really nice to see you, but it's a hotel where you can go to Junom.

First phrase phrases can be deleted:

• I'll pick something up/drink something.
• If you need to get out of the balcony, pay attention to the details.
• May I meet you in Charlie.
• I need to leave.

In each case, the number of people to choose from is one of them. The most common types of problems are the nature of the problem and not the problem.

Complete exercises 56 and 57.

4.6. Compliments

For many people use the "create property" and "create property" associations associated with the ability and the value

2756 65

critique and deal with conflicts. It is not for the purpose of acknowledging the validity of the deletion of compliments. The tradition of the socio-phobia of Neredko is a matter of trust with the team. They prefer not to compliment, fearing that this could lead to "unpredictable" reactions (including positive ones) that they feel they won't be able to handle.

People immediately voice criticism when they notice wrong behavior, but often forget to praise someone who deserves it, although praise is more conducive to interaction than criticism.

If you have any issues with this, please feel free to contact me for more information.

Compliment model

1. Explain your similarity:
• "I think you are the one who slipped",
• "I think you are a good poet",
- "I ch i i yu yu yu to..." »» »".

2. Support the following steps:
• "I think you are the one who slipped",

• "I think you are a good poet",
- "I ch i i yu yu yu to..." »» »".
3. Find out what exactly you have been told:
• "I think you are the one who slipped",
• "I think you are a good poet",
- "I ch i i yu yu yu to..." »» »".

This is the model you are referring to as a complimenting artist. It is recommended that you pay attention to the possibilities of these extravagant compliments. These simple compliments can also be evaluated by the user. In the case of a successful compliment, postmodern on this scheme, it will not have a proper setting.

Complete the task 58.

66

These are used in model design, displaying the ability to create compliments. Perhaps it is possible to distinguish between those who are unseen, those who are unseen. This is an actual job that will work. Certainly, this particular approach does not cover the same, and although there are many people who want to share the compliments of this. No new practices have been announced that your new sample will not be able to save any and all of them spontaneously. Good practice is to make sure that you get the most out of it. All of these are likely to be available in a variety of ways.

And do not hesitate to compliment each compliment.

Complete the task 59.

Commemoration of the name of a compliment

It's a sociophobia that threatens to compliment compliments. They are supposed to protect the script. For example, when they hear a compliment about their new clothes, they respond, "That was the cheapest," to good singing, "My voice doesn't really fit that song," to a good speech, "I've lost my way up a few times."

When it comes to complimenting the best compliments and looking after them, it's a very nice and comfortable place for us.

How to properly compliment compliments

Publish files (thank you, very nice, that you have taken a note and etc.), make sure you remember your name. You can not find the page you are looking for.

Note: • «Great space. It's a dummy, it's not working well ».

67

• «A mile away from your pages, which you have already covered. This is a very simple product that is not designed to work ».

Complete exercises 60 and 61.

4.7. Thank you very much

If you are a social traveler who wants to get married to him or her. This is a description of a different category: if you want to specify the output, then the page, then the second one will be displayed. Poetry about the subject in which you will receive a slave. What is the best way to go about it?

Ideal design model

1. Make sure you have something in store for you.
2. Presented in the following form in the form of a positive prediction, namely:

- "I would like to...",
- "I want...",
- "I would be grateful if...",
- "I want to ask you about...",
- "I would prefer that..."

As you can see, the most important part of this

process is the ability to communicate with the developer. The process of selecting the validity of the sample, the number of which, which you are looking for, the number of wasted was completed. Share: "Can't you just drop me off?" and "I though, what you're getting rid of". Or: "Can't you just get rid of this mess?" and "I though, you've been awarded this job".

3. Make sure you are clear and concrete. Someone to say goodbye to, let alone know from here:

- "I However, what you are trying to do is not save it".
- "I have a hotel, which I have up to 10 times".

68

4. Do not waste words, just translate your words: clear, clear, clear, clear. For example, it's not a good idea to say "In the case of luxury, you may not have a problem with 10. It is not possible to remember it."

5. There are not many things that you can do to get rid of them. The number of applications that you do not have is one of the most popular. Nikoda does not specify a double-entry price. In other words, you don't have to say, "Because otherwise I'm going to be very nervous, and I've been very tired lately, and you don't have to do that to your friends, I'm always calling anyway..."

6. Offer another key to your job. Note: "I'm trying to figure out what I'm looking for in an episode of this week. Do you sleep? » or: «If a hotel chooses to buy a book on this site: in the cinema, in the theater or in a new book. Do you remember me? »

This model is suitable for your situation, which is what you are talking about, what you are talking about. In the current situation, the most important thing is that when it comes down to it, the official tone of the case will be clear. In the most recent situations you can enter and enter:

• Are you not interested in having a rejuvenated bed?
• Leave, sketch.
• The whole of Mandarin wood, which is well known.

And do not forget that what you are looking for is a well-formatted version of what you want to do.

Complete exercises 62 and 63.

4.8. Rating

If it's what you're trying to do, you're not going to think it's not 'what you want to share, it's not you. It's sociophobic that it's hard to say 'not'. They

A positive reaction is needed, which is not to mention a risky decision. As a result, we are not able to find out what we are looking for in other countries, which is a source of frustration and frustration. The poem is one of the most important.

You can change your mouse, display the strokes displayed on the screen, return to level 3. When selecting the range, do not.

Model «ideal design»

1. Find a place where you can get something done. Tell a friend who you are.
2. Formulate your outcome in terms of positive and positive behaviors, as well as other things that you can do.
3. For such a decision, do not use any additional prints. The number of applications that can be defined as "not" does not have a fixed number of prints.
4. Do not use slides, which indicate your output: deceptive, possible, random, smooth. Add: "I'm clearly not a bidder" and "No, I'm not a bitch".
5. You can, however, not agree to disagreements.

Note:

*Stefan:*You can easily find this book. Can or should you

like it?

*Category:*No, Stephen, I'm not a big fan of books, but I'm so obsessed with many things. If you are interested in this topic, please contact us today.

*Rooms:*Can't you just load and unzip menus? Adrian: There is no such thing as a city in that peak. Why do you not pay attention to what you do?

*Ted:*What do you want to do next? Paula: None.

70

Please note that this is not the case, it is not specified, what you are doing is not specified. Note: "I really like it, well ..."

If you are unable to find the "no" option, then you will not be able to find the one you are trying to use. Note: "I do not know. X hotel o u o u..... Is it possible that you are going to sleep? » This is because the time is required to create a "no" position, or not. If you are looking for "da", this is the name of the most trusted item.

Exercises 64 and 65.

4.9. How to react to an issue

The traditional sociophobia is to express your views and views, whichever you choose, which will not be noticed.

Ideal model

1. Download this item to your friends (run par).
2. Note the value of the second keystroke.
3. On the possibility of alternative alternatives.

Primers (Rationale 5.8):

*Stefan:*Well, you can definitely get this one straight. Of course, you do not have to worry about it, as long as you do it. If it's enough, we can change the range.

*Rooms:*It is necessary to have a crane, as is often the case. I do not think your review is a bad one for a drug addict. Is it possible to work on the page, or do you want to save it?

*Ted:*Hall. Is it possible, in another case?

71

What kind of behavior do you expect to find in this case?

In another case, if you do not agree with the refusal (for example, when communicating with a seller or an official), you can repeat your request with slight variations, trying to express it in clearer and more understandable language.

Note:

- I'm a hotel to save your mail on the new home project. Do you need an address?
- You can do this, sir, or just leave.
- But when it comes to telephone scales, it can be used in any type of working day. When it comes to hotels, you're the one who's registered.
- You have never been informed, sir. We will build all the rooms.
- is not able to expose to the poll. This is because of the lack of personal information on this site, but it is important to note that we do not have any information about it.
- It is not possible to delete this item.
- It is not uncommon for wine to be consumed. And the most successful attempt to solve a problem - it's my ability to register.
- Well, let's say this in video clips.

Exercises 66 and 67.

4.10. Review critique

One of the most important things that can happen to a reporter is to read his critique. This is because it has the ability to select different types of files, which are

stored in the folder for which you are browsing. This is a chrome finish, which is a great addition to your wardrobe.
This is a sociophobic tradition, which is believed to criticize others, which is why it is not uncommon for them to be criticized.
72
try the ability of aggression, which you have not been able to overcome. This poem does not seem to be the only version of its critique.
How do you read good reviews?
1. Determine what you want to cover.
2. Create it for yourself.
3. Distinguish between the concrete and the concrete, which distinguishes your critique and in which it is acknowledged.
4. One should not criticize one of these positions.
5. Do not use slogans, which can describe your critique: deceptive, powerful, honest, clever.
6. Do not mention any of the criticisms of your critique.
7. Provide alternate solutions for troubleshooting problems.
8. Provide your own ability to react to your critique.
Note:
• «I want to add your watch to the watch. This is the one with the saddle and the one. In the next race, you will be punctual ».
• "I do not know where the cellular view is located on the TV. It's impossible to log. I recommend to turn off the TV on the screen 10 times a week. What are you looking for? »
• I in fact, it is not a very good thing that you are referring to the translation of Roman and Veri, which

is not predestined. C is not a free data center. However, it is also a matter of time and importance, as it is not possible for you to get rid of it, we do not need it at all. What are you talking about? »

It is important to critique the way things are done, if you are willing to share and support your social contacts. Normally you can easily get rid of clutter you don't need. If you do not have the ability to write a critique, it will be the same as the one that will not be able to retrieve it.

73

This item is subject to change or any further frustration.

Execution critique - we do not have a social right. If you want to get rid of clutter, you should try to get rid of any clutter you may have.

Note that what you are looking for is a good way to get rid of clutter you do not need. Your reaction will not be positive, nor will it be a pity, and you will miss out on a new form of education.

Exercises 68 and 69.

4.11. Reaction to criticism

As a result, the critique of this matter is confirmed by the automation bases. No response has been received to the response to any criticism at your address. It's not uncommon for people to throw a stone at your garden in response ("But are you new..."), try to absolve themselves of blame ("I had no choice because..."), or start arguing with you ("You can I make a kimim-nibudud delam, if I want to date", "Can I send something to you?

Possible reactions show the increase in size and not the size of the situation.

Model of an ideal approach to critique:
1. Subscribe to your news items.
*2. Summarize*There are many other types of tools that you can use to get rid of clutter you need.
3. Submit your comments to critics.
74
Primer predisposition that you are looking for or your alternative prediction.
Primers (Rationale 5.10):
• "I am very low. Itak, where did you get the redemption? You can use all of them. There are no entries or entries in the page ".
• «Drugs, I do not know, because many things do not work for me. Just for menus on the channel - a wonderful tool for communication. Can I have a new one * while watching TV, and do I have to wait? »
• "I recommend, that you sport this week. I want to give you a good price, well, of course, you're trying to get it home. I've presiding over. Who do we sleep with?
Remember that you will achieve great results in your reaction to criticism if you work effectively with your negative thoughts, as suggested in Chapter 3. If criticism of your insignificant act causes you to think that the other person completely rejects you, it is natural that on the other hand, sliding on the "ideal behavior" screen will cause a lot of problems.
Complete tasks 70 and 71.
4.12. Chaplaincy to Social Words
This is a case in point, and there are a number of issues that have been raised in the past. If you want to complete all the puzzles, you will get the desired effect from the niche. For this purpose, you will find automation tips that will help you improve your daily

program. It is very important that you regularly check what you are looking for and what you are trying to do.

5. Addition of attachments

5.1. Chemistry will unravel

In this case, you will definitely need to work on the situation, which is a very long-term solution. The current situation is always reflected in the distribution of information. This is unnecessary. However, it is possible for you to make sure that you get the most out of your phone. There are many things to do in this regard. The people who watch the TV show are the ones who make the most of the news or even the newspaper quotes. Special audio recorders are provided with music, which can be used to record music.

5.2. Protective woodworking

Now that you have learned to change your thoughts to more rational ones, already know how to relax quickly and effectively, and have practiced a large number of social skills, you are ready to gradually come face to face with situations that cause you anxiety.

The strength of social situations can be enhanced by the results of your work with the tools and skills. Well, it's possible that you're going to be severely annoyed by one or two other situations.

Creating and retrieving the location of a file that is used to retrieve data from a location or location. Other languages, in the "persevere" section of your trip.

This is the head of the group, which we all preach. In fact, it is the same as the one on the other, and it is the most important of all. Gala 5 course, where is this

the structure of the menu is slow. When you work, you

follow the principle of principle: "I like a rope, it works like a bear".

We do not use all the tools that allow you to maximize the effect of the application, which will not work.

5.3. Production of check cards for rehearsals

Causes of cracking occur on the part of the effect, which is a bit of a good idea.

We do not use a lot of cards, which we do not use for each other. The logo, the numbers from 0 to 100, need to be carefully selected, as well as the value of the item, which shows the value of the unit.

Note:

• Whip coffee in your work environment with your colleges. (70)

• Download the "private" item, if you want to go to the movie. (30)

You can deal with a lot of great cards. We will be able to work with more than one of the most popular on the market.

Determine the number of cards that are located in the situation. For easy situations, it may be necessary to have a separate card, which can be used to extend the distance between the steps.

Note:

Situation: Drink coffee.

1. Make coffee from the plastic stacks of guests in our house. (40).

2. Place coffee on plastic wrap in a jar of other seeds. (50)

77

3. Make coffee from a lollipop with sugar in the room at home. (65).

4. Make coffee from a loaf of sugar in a jar of other seeds. (75)

5. Make coffee from a sugar cane on a workbench. (80)

Situation: Find out more about submissions.

1. Share this libo with your work colleagues. (40)
2. Select "I do not agree with ..." on the job directory. (60)
3. Distribute this book to the working staff. (70)
4. Select "I do not agree with ..." the workload of the staff. (80)

All cards in the shopping cart are listed by you, but you will not be able to return them. When you try out all the cards, the problem of your sociophobia is different.

Certainly well-groomed shades, suitable for exercise, which are very comfortable for you.

Complete the challenge 72.

5.4. Scheduling planning

These are all card types that are sorted by location and location.

Indeed, the practice of recruiting on a regular basis is more or less straightforward. Many applications are threaded and receive neutral energy. Practice shows: you should try to get the most out of it, you should try to find one. Delete, if any, you want to get rid of clutter. Washing hands - This is a ball bearing the shape of the ballot box and the position of the ballot box.

For example, you can save up to 200 points. If the result is an extension of up to 220 points, the level at which you enter your cell is:

78

• Reassign this note in the same time as the match submission.

• Promote the college to program the most.

- Post a check at the shopping center.
- List checks in most supermarkets.

You can add one or more tools. Complete the task 73.

5.5. How to complete the challenge

Try levels 3, 4, 5, etc., even if you have completed the challenge. One of the most important methods of analysis is the implementation of various procedures, which are displayed in each appraisal. This procedure enables us to measure all the trials of mycelium on this specific situation.

This "proprietary" option may be related to the number of issues in the application, which is not the same. In each case, you have to make sure that all the information you provide is up to you.

You pay attention to each situation, which is a detailed description of the milk supply. Please be aware that you are in this situation. Be realistic and rational. In other words, draw yourself how each person at a party will think that you are beautiful, and even better imagine how after the conversation with one person is over, you will be looking for someone else to talk to.

Help us to complete the challenge, to relax and to make it easier to get along, it's easy to do.

You need to specify the completion of each exercise. Please note that it is necessary to make an application that does not contain any of the items that are needed.

79

For the best results, you can try again. Any application you need to complete at least three sizes. Only those who have been tested and those who have been shown what they are, can be either.

Be sure to save your most recent results. It's worth noting that you'll be able to fill in the blanks that you want to create. For example, if you want to get rid of all the clutter you have with the Ulysses and get rid of it, it's a hurricane or a hurricane.

Complete the task 74.

5.6. Special Tasting: "Win a Narrow"

This is a sociophobic tradition that strives to write your message and the character of each character, as if he or she were different. It is very important that you do not store any items and, if necessary, that you do not need anything from them. If they think that they are sweating now, they constantly wipe themselves with a handkerchief, look at the floor, find an excuse to refuse the offered tea, hide their features under a thick layer of cosmetics. The result is that it does not contain anything that is not enough, if you do not want to use this "problem". All existing streams will not be able to support any situation in which traffic can not be supported. The streaming screen displays the message, even if it has been displayed silently, which displays the name of the item. He,

One of the most important things to do is to close the jar - to make sure that other types of vinegar are present or that are present. Other languages, "save money". For example, you can choose which one is the same as the one or the other. Copy, download easily

80

gromco, which would otherwise be omitted: "Oh no, open this door. This is a continuous increase. Wertowski is annoying."

This is a very difficult task, because the task is very clear and difficult to control. It is the same as the practice of trying to find a negative message about them. With different pages, it is possible that you will find them, which will be used by the media.

The most important set for you, which you have defined as your developer strategy, which is your personal favorite style. The layout shows: it is possible to separate only the first stroke, and then all the layers are smooth and smooth.

As a rule, you should be able to sort your problems with flash drives. Of course, whatever happens, the reaction of the people will not be negative, as it may be that they are with you.

All you have to do is submit a plan of construction to the people who have been to each other, who will be able to find you. This logo, which you will practice on your own, is what you will find on the site.

Many applications from the 3-year-old list of "high-yield" products, and you can do the same: are you there or what? If this is something you are working on, you should try to find out if there are any issues that you may have.

This will support this application for this purpose, which will be practiced in this case.

Complete the task 75.

5.7. Additional tasks

If you have completed the application program, it can be tried, depending on whether you want to add one or more of the additional values. You can take advantage of the situation you are in and then give yourself a chance to get rid of some of the problems. Each pair of shoes, which you can try, smo-

If you want to get out of a situation where you have a lot of problems or just want to get rid of it. You will need to check the availability of the contents of the game.

Resolve the default application, selecting the value of each item.

• Store in the store stores and files, first and foremost, do not buy.

• Go to the best car in the yard, get the car you are looking for.

• Can or should not be used for any purpose.

• Mention the number of messages sent or received by other users.

• Find a restaurant without cosmetics.

• Release for store-bought packages, save what you have lost, or get lost.

• Only display items in the window, which can be stored in the store.

• Check by phone at the cuckoo-level check box and in the list of each number do not specify the number of entries.

• Open immediately to a restaurant restaurant without a hitch.

• Protect files that you can print, but not selected.

• Spot on a file or code in the file.

• Buy money, books or other items.

• List officers in the restaurant branch, which are all listed.

• Select comma-nibudn au poshndno vecheroom.

• Select what you do not want and do not want to share.

• Check all names, brochures: books, bicycles, bank accounts, bottles of mineral water and water. d.

82

Rejoice in these prophecies, you can say: "This is a blasphemy, it is not a pity! It's not something to share ».

It is very important that you understand the meaning

of what you mean when it comes to what you look for in yourself. We need a lot of people to check and check that you are not saving any cookies.
Develop ideas, developed in this format, for new wash cards as well as the application of the 72 and one item.
5.8. Possible difficulties
by default search prompt
A) If the application is used correctly.
If you do not want to fill out the form below, as you are currently viewing this page, you can pre-select the following:
• Distribute new cards with promotional features, such as those with a great deal of support. We can create beautiful objects, primer, chisel prismatic people, male or female, female or male. If you want to change the following: first, create a neutral version and every page you want to read.
• Try, be proud of yourself and be your friend. Analyze your missiles, the most common triangular trials and tribulations. If you do not have one, you will be presented with the 3rd grade. If you are not in a position to play on level 4.
B) If the application is not modified.
If you do not want to delete this message, you will be prompted to complete the application, in which case you will need to read the following:
b *
83
• Are you aware of the connection between your and your trip? For example, when completing an application - visit the company. Most of all that can be found, which is what you are looking for, and you will not be able to find one. If you do not have a clear password, you may need to worry about what is going

on. In the case of a slider that slides, the new card is displayed:

• Are there any new provocative trials of mysticism, published in the context of this trial, which are not in the process of being developed? If this is the case, you should close the table for analysis of the mouse and try it yourself, and if you do not find one.

Q) If you are interested in the reactions of other people.

One of the things you and other people can do is keep up the good content. It is recommended that you simply create a cache of the contents of the file, and then select the one you want to use. Possibly, on your password this one reads: "What are you talking about?" or "Do not hurt me!". This allows you to update your trip. Poetry in the doldrums, which you can see in your trip in this situation.

We are constantly updating, which by analyzing the various possibilities of negative reactions will be discussed. You presume that the negative result is not serious, as you can see the previous one, and each one. You will be determined by the most positive position. The negative reaction is one of the emerging ones. In this case, you should change the idea that a negative reaction means a negative attitude towards you personally (see Logical Fallacy 4 in Chapter 3), or that if someone has a negative opinion of you, then it is a complete tragedy (smog logical version 5 in level 3).

84

5.9. Planning social contacts

All of the above are specific to what you are looking for. It results in the fulfillment of the status quo in our current social situations.

Lots of people, traditional sociophobia, sometimes have a very different kind of Druze and sometimes enjoy socializing. It is not possible to claim that this is a non-profit initiative, which can be used as part of social work.

We've a primer. It is possible, as you may see, that the full-fledged custom-based systems of your contacts. The "Druze Dose" option states that the key contains the level of the tree, which is related to the size of the connection. We recommend that you check with them, who will help and support new developments. You will be able to see where all the social news videos are and how many trips there are.

Suggestions include social media contacts. Think about people who are talking about each other or their names. If so, we will work with you. On the other hand, there are times when we are in your school, in your school, in the club, in the club, and so on. d.

You can select the intensity of your contact with each other, set a new range, and even if you are one of them. d.

You do not know where you are going to go, you do not know where you are going to get what you want.

Complete the task 76.

It is not uncommon for a person to have a concussion when it comes to exercise. There are some of them that are most useful for completing the most recent exercises that you need to find in the "Candidates" section. You can create, copy, and paste in cocoa-

nibble club. Choose one or more clubs that reflect your interests, for example, a club of amateur photographers, nature lovers, a sports club, a society of theater lovers, a dance group. This information can be used in most domicile cultures or in the Soviet Union.

There are many ways to increase your ability to work. This is what cocaine is all about. Support the activity of club clubs, institute or maintenance, the speed of the flash on the deck (first, if you want to take them). Make sure you get the latest news from hotels near you. There is no such thing as a post office. We will work with you to find the right solution.

Complete the task 77.

All of these can be used to protect the most common of these diseases. Note that this type of necrotic ermine will make you feel bad about all the blemishes and blemishes you have to deal with.

5.10. Program Evaluation

It's you who tried all the tricks, filled out a lot of challenges. This is all about freebies.

This is not a connector yet. To strengthen and increase your achievements, you need to regularly return to the "Theoretical Book" and "Workbook", read, analyze, plan exercises and perform them.

Boilers that can be shared are free of charge, without any additional requirements. You regularly check your psychotherapist's views. Of course, this is a simple reminder of the results of your search.

Distinguish between the balloon team, named after us in round 2.

86

Exercises 78, 79 and 80.

You can observe the effect of completing programs such as your psychotherapist and get rid of the problem in that part.

Suggestions for advanced features:

• In the case of unsolicited plans, you may be working

on a detailed plan.

• There are many symphobic symphobia clues. We need to take more intensive courses in psychotherapy. Explain this ability to your psychotherapist. This tag can be used to print a medical record.

• Many may not have any symptoms that are not related to the sociophobia that are affected by the lesions. Exploit this is your psychotherapist.

Try your mouse to get rid of your psychotherapist.

This is the best TRADE STAGE

DENVITE OUT

Date	Attentio n	Poster value	Excerpts	Excerpts	For zemetok

91

PROFESSIONALS

Exercise 1

Record your name and the date of the work on the "Work in Tradition" page.

Operate on page 6. Complete the first update. This day, you will definitely need to record everything that you are looking for in the program. These are referred to in section 1.5 "Theoretical books".

Exercise 2

Check out what you are talking about, as it is possible for you to be the most successful person in this program.

If you want to get rid of clutter you don't need, and try to get rid of clutter.

Get rid of clutter you don't need, and you can also swipe it and swipe it.

If you want, you can find yourself a second assistant, for example, if the assistant you choose will not be able to constantly help you or if it will be difficult for him alone to cope with this work.

RATATE: How Much Support Do You Have: ____________________

The ones that can be used in the "Theoretical books" category, but do not include any of them. The keys do not quote the key 2.

***Proofreading*3**

If you prefer, as you would like to know the theory, you will find out about the latest developments. Please note, do not delete-

92

or in a theoretical game. Verify the passwords, prevent the page, and delete your passwords. We invite you to read some interesting stories.

In the case of accidental headaches, one of the variants may be different. All you have to do is select the one you are looking for.

1. This is a sociophobic tradition, as follows:
(a) reviews of other countries;
(b) averaging other large numbers of people;
in) a home in the center of women; d) public goodies.

2. This is a sociophobic tradition, the following:
a) create a very interesting app in many societies various situations;
b) overcome the social situation of the child, the child is possible;
(v) in the situation of the establishment of such a branch, which
extract negative products;
(g) points (a), (b) and ()).

3. Maintenance:
a) it is a common notion of sociophobia;
b) is one of sociophobic videos;
c) concludes that what one is trying to do is to lose;
g) not a syllable, as sociophobia.

4. You can use a dialect, a traditional sociophobic, by:
(a) such as;
(b) that which has a beautiful crown;
(v) the number of submissions;
g) this nickname does not vary; all items are included.

5. Sociophobia:
a) Reduces the yield: 0.05% of the yield is high;
93
(b) it is generally associated with the existence of other types of solids;
in) it excels in secondary school; (d) you have a lot of good professions.

Reviews on postings and postings in the name

Call 1

1a. It does not appear to be unobtrusive, nor is it the same and not the most luxurious. Situations in which the site does not appear to be open show no traffic.

16. PROVIDED.

1c. This item may not be on sale, but will not be replaced.

1g. This is related only to those who share their views on sociophobic videos.

If you have never been to a party before, check out 2.1.

Call 2

2a. That's fine, not bad.

26. This is exactly what was going on.

2c. This is exactly what was going on.

2g. PROVIDED.

If you have never been to a party before, check out 2.1.

Vopros 3

Yes. INVOLVED. 36. INVOLVED. .B. INVOLVED. .G. PROVIDED.

It is possible, however, to associate it with trivia, whether or not the situation is different and whether it is true or not.

If you have never been to a party before, check out 2.1.

94

Vopros 4

4a. INVOLVED. Smotri p. (g).

46. INVOLVED. Many people are born without a trip.

4c. INVOLVED. This message does not appear to be a response, but it does not appear.

4g. PROVIDED.

If you have never been to a party before, check out 2.1.

Vopros 5

5a. INVOLVED. Out of 3 to 13%, that is, they are sociophobic and have one in their life, at a time when 1-2.5% are in the market.

56. INVOLVED. Extension of publicity and publicity with the most important thing of the day.

5c. INVOLVED. The sociophobia that pervades each of the 15th and 20th centuries.

5g. PROVIDED.

If you have never been to a party before, check out 2.1.

Procedure 3 (Proposition)

6. Sociophobia can be viewed:

(a) the level of public outcry;

(b) the number of letters in the subdivision and the subdivisions

European;

(vi) copying of other goods by road;

g) the hormonal trend in puberty.

7. Sociophobia can be as follows:

(a) in support of specific therapies or drugs;

b) non-alcoholic;

(v) only medical comments;

g) with the help of appropriate therapies.

95

8. Occupational therapy:

(a) Orientation on the validation of symptoms;

(b) renewal of domestic contracts;

(v) kept in the analysis of the prospectus;

(g) points (a) and (b) prevail.

9. Occupational therapy in sociophobia:

(a) does not contain anything related to mycelium

analysis;
(b) focus only on social security contributions
weeks;
in) * encloses the provision of related data;
g) indicates the failure of the department and many do not believe
or another.

Reviews and offers (promotion)

Vopros 6

Ba. Inevitably. There is no such thing as trauma or sociophobia.
Bb. Inevitably. The availability of letters in the guipure of the present predominates only as a possible factor.
bv. That's right. The imitation of the societal phobias of the nobility as a result of the veritable ability
Bg. Inevitably. Some of the key elements of the Hormonal status can be defined as possible.
If you find yourself in a situation like this, see section 2.2.

Vopros 7

7a. That's right. This has been done several times.
76. Unpredictably.
7c. Inevitably. Pre-treatment therapy can be specially primed without licorice.
7g. Inevitably. Medical treatment without the specific therapies that can be effective.
If you have never found one, please refer to section 2.3.

96

Vopros 8

8a. That's right. 86. Okay.
8c. Inevitably. Analyzing the proposed version does not make it difficult.
8g. Okay (this is a nice quote).

If you have not heard of it yet, please note section 2.3.
Call 9
9a. Inevitably. One of the most popular therapies in the field - working with the development of a tree.
96. Unpredictable. The promotion of social justice - only one of the aspirations of successive therapies.
9c. That's right. Occupational therapy all encompasses the application of the previous application.
9g. Inevitably. Detailed planning is very important in real estate. It's worth noting that it's a real bargaining chip. Analysis and preparation of provocative trials of different types of cases.
If you have any questions, please feel free to share your information. If you want to get rid of clutter you don't need, we recommend you go back to level 2, step 2.3. We've got to see some issues.
If you want to change the text of the text and the correct wording of the process, you can use the 2.4 version.

Exercise 4.

Test Leibovich (translation result)

You will need an entry for 24 situations. Some unscrupulous people are aware of the common problems of the day.
Suggest, depending on whether you are in the current situation or whether you have (in the case of a case), a number of cases.
7 - 2756
97
1 - no transport;
2 - light rail;
3 - commuter train;
4 - Intensive travel.
To find out what steps you are going to take or what

you are looking for in a 4-ball scale situation:
1 - nicoda (0%);
2 - content (1 - 33%);
3 - share (34 - 67%);
4 - fixed (68 - 100%).

Diagnostics

1. Phone coverage in the application of other solutions. 12 3 4 1234
2. Training in a new group. 1234 1234
3. Work on chairs. 12 3 4 12 3 4
4. Whip a cup of coffee in the cafeteria most of the time. 1234 1234
5. Composition with the most popular Lithuanian / Chinese. 12 3 4 1234
6. Public deployment. 12 3 4 12 3 4
7. Get on the road. 12 3 4 12 3 4
8. Reload the job after loading another key. 1234 1234
9. Delete entries in postal records. 12 3 4 12 3 4
10. Remove the small bowl. 12 3 4 12 3 4
11. Be careful with chemistry. 12 3 4 12 3 4
12. The number of people who are illegitimate. 12 3 4 12 3 4
13. Delivery of private toilets. 12 3 4 12 3 4
14. Vote in the municipality, in which you will find the site. 12 3 4 12 3 4
15. Switch to the center of calls. 12 3 4 12 3 4
16. Without prejudice to the word "submission". 12 3 4 1234
17. Examination of practical or legal documents. 1234 1234

98

18. Release your unobstructed or uninsulated windows, which are slightly damaged. 12 3 4 12 3 4
19. Display the amount of liquid in the glass. 1234

1234

20. Group documents in groups. 12 3 4 12 3 4

21. Introduce romantic or sexual norms. 12 3 4 12 3 4

22. Enter items in a magazine (with the same date as the date). 12 3 4 1234

23. Build a vault. 12 3 4 12 3 4

24. Determine the location of the Commercial Agent. 12 3 4 1234

Sell your items in all 24 situations: first item - the value of your items, the value - the level of the situation. Download the most recent results:

Business Rating: ___________________________________

Situation Rating: _________________________

General image type: ______________________________

Exercise 5.
Personal test situation

These are just some of the things that we can do to help you find the right place for you. This can be a situation where you can get rid of it from a different point of view.

You define situations based on the following principle: "If I cope with these situations and do not experience tension in them, then I will no longer have Secrets of Social phobia." Other languages, do not select situations, which are stored in the window, do not have any names (if any).

Situations that are different in terms of possibilities are very detailed. Other languages, not "select code-nibud", and "connect to" Belize Orel "

7 *

99

with ». As you can see, we can easily find out about the situation. We also need to find out the specifics, specifics and the best possible situations. If possible, try to find the right one, not the most common one in this situation. It is possible that you will find out what the situations are when completing the challenge 4.

Note that these are not unique to each situation ("Specify the number of rows and Themes"), as well as which one.

What a great idea:

- Visits to another (as well as to whom?).
- Store this item in a magazine (in which one?).
- • Reassembles of auto-recovery or recovery.
- Sit in the prime (in which?).
- Serve at a restaurant (as well as with us?).
- Find places on the road (in which? Which?) And all

the places you are looking for.

- Mail the envelope to the mail.
- Whip up a cup of coffee in a coffee shop.
- Execute with a request or a lesson (where? Will I return?)
- Select in the search box (what? Button?).

Increase situations between 1 and 5 numbers.

Let's give you a break, and you'll be welcomed in these situations. For this, use an 8-ball scale, which is 1 - a cocoa-free volley, and 8 - a full panicle. Unleash and recite in the jar the new figure, giving you the support you need. For example, if you are in a situation where you have a bad one, you have "easy disks" (2), or you have a "blue one" (4).

1

012345678

You are comfortable (0). Cocoa-libo volleyballs (1). Nebulous discomforts (2). Cylindrical disc comfort (3).

100

Distinctively nervous (4). Appearance recording (5). Exercise pressure (6). Power train (7). Full panic (8).

2____

____

012345678

You are comfortable (0). Cocoa-libo volleyballs (1). Nebulous discomforts (2). Cylindrical disc comfort (3). Distinctively nervous (4). Appearance recording (5). Exercise pressure (6). Power train (7). Full panic (8).

3____

____

012345678

You are comfortable (0). Cocoa-libo volleyballs (1). Nebulous discomforts (2). Cylindrical disc comfort (3). Distinctively nervous (4). Appearance recording (5).

Exercise pressure (6). Power train (7). Full panic (8).

4

012345678

You are comfortable (0). Cocoa-libo volleyballs (1). Nebulous discomforts (2). Cylindrical disc comfort (3). Distinctively nervous (4). Appearance recording (5). Exercise pressure (6). Power train (7). Full panic (8).

5

012345678

You are comfortable (0). Cocoa-libo volleyballs (1). Nebulous discomforts (2). Cylindrical disc comfort (3). Distinctively nervous (4). Appearance recording (5).

Exercise pressure (6). Power train (7). Full panic (8).

Submit items in the video below:

DATE _________ OBJECTIVES ___________________

This test situation can be used to distribute the effectiveness of your work with sociophobia.

The sequels, which are also used in Exercise 5, can be used as "Theoretical books".

Exercise 6

InThere are not many prime ministers who divide themselves, that they may be rich, that they may prosper, and that they may prosper. Unpredictable charts distinguish the point, the punctuation - the number, and the number of points.

"I'm definitely nervous. This is the content of the message. It's good that I'm not getting any money. You will be able to qualify as a candidate. It's a scale that needs to be glorified. I will be with the same age as the year and to the body of the company to the soi of the usual clothes. This will allow you to clear the door. That's great. Sorry, this is a crackdown. What I mean is ".

Show regular items.

Provisional items in practice 6

Submit a message, send us a free script, send a message without any change.

"I'm definitely nervous. This is the content of the message. It's good that I'm not getting any money. You will be able to qualify as a candidate. It's a scale that needs to be glorified. I'll be in my best weekend commmim, year ka ka

102

companies in your own addition. This will allow you to download files.

That's great. Sorry, this is a crackdown. What I mean is ".

Release moments:

•The phrase "I do not know what I mean" is a myth, as it were. The results are: in this case, they are not valid (and possibly: this will be a disaster). It is possible to use this tool to drive the truck.

• The phrase “You will not be able to qualify as a candidate” will be deleted as a result, depending on what you are doing.

• The phrase "Sorry, you're going to crash" will be deleted as soon as possible. One thing is clear from this, which is a concrete piece of clothing dressed as a "raskis". Anything else on this site can help you find the right one. Other languages, this is a missile.

If you want to get rid of clutter you need to scroll down to the 3.1 and 3.2 range, and then select 6.

Exercise 7

This is an example of a 6-year-old girl who has been around for some time.

Subject	

Love	
Mysli	

103

View text and delete the previous one in the form: "I am Tak schastliv. Submit a message directly. They will allow you to save your mail for 10 minutes. I do not think it is worthwhile to spend on such items. . I'm sure they'll put me in."

Describe the current situation, even the formality of the analysis of the missile.

I feel like my throat is sieving. From the two pillows, perched on the roof of the house, each one was made of silver. I'm shooting a lot of them ».

Subject	
Love	
Mysli	

Protect page and view custom items.

Provisional items on sale7

Subject	The message is sent for 10 minutes.
Love	You.
Mysli	Submit a message directly. I do not think it is worthwhile to spend on such items. Oh dear, that's what I mean.
Subject	From the two pillows, perched on the top of the pillars, take all the linen.

Love	Pechal.
Mysli	I'm shooting a lot of money.

If you do not have any issues with this topic, you will need to select level 3 from each item, if any.
104

Exercise 8

Divide companies, cities and municipalities, separate forms for the second half of the situation:
"I'm all right, as far as I can tell." I'm sorry, you've been screwed. If you want to get rid of clutter you may not be able to get enough of it. . Polish neurotics. There are no such thing as a new home. The menu is silently loading ».

Subject	
Love	
Mysli	

"I'm a checher bubet kaestroph. I'm getting lost. This is a beautiful post on the floor! They know about the kilometer. It is recommended that you do not have to spend a fortune on spider mites. I'm very nervous, but I'm not happy to tell you what I mean by coffee. It's your own career ».

Subject	
Love	

Mysli	

Experienced activities in practice 8

Subject	(Duma om etom) An acquaintance with Harry.
Love	Travel.
Mysli	I'm sorry, you've been screwed. You will not be able to find anything similar to me. . Polish neurotics. There are no such thing as a new home.

105

Subject	Price on the backrest. The waitress in the cafe.
Love	Travel, nervousness.
Mysli	This is a disaster. I'm getting lost. Get information on mileage. We do not know where to place the wine in the cafe.

If you do not have access to the freebies, you may need to enter the "Theoretical book" as the number of items that you have.

Exercise 9

Release situations from your previous plan and immediately move to new locations, cities and municipalities.

Subject	
Love	
Mysli	

If you do not have the required permissions on the previous page, you will not need it. Refer to "Theoretical book" and provide information.

Exercise 10

You will be able to create new positions by completing the 9: Exercise Forms Intention Form and Reconstruction.

There are no standard entries yet. The most important thing you can do is to try to fill out the form below.

Examination &

InComplete form that you need to update and distribute:

106

Subject	Ball in the mix of flavors.
Love	I remember that he was not found (100%).
Mysli	I can not pay (100%). It is said that nervousness is associated with overeating (90%).

Your variant of filling out forms:

Subject	
Love	
Mysli	

Regular answers in Exercise 11:

Subject	Dinner.
Love	Download (80).

Mysli	I did not like it (80). If you do not find the link you are looking for then just select a Druze (75). I need to find a job (90).

Announcements:

• "Mishloach bullet" is displayed, as is the case with the MIXED MONUMENTS step, level 80.

• The phrase "I do not understand" is the result of a change in the nature of the study. This is not allowed to display in the table.

• The phrase "I've nervous about the most important things" is a general, not a current one.

• The message "If you do not have a message that you do not have a Druid" or "I do not want to send it to anyone". The "I do not need" message can not be displayed on the screen.

Exercise 12

Explain the need for a situation in which you are dealing with different circumstances.

107

Repair molds, dry cleaning materials and other solvents. By default, you will be able to increase the intensity of the activity and the percentage of activity that you have.

Date	
Subject	
Love	
Mysli	

Try to fill out the form below form:

1. Project management - is it something concrete and objective, or a mix of goals, money, ideas or business? What did it look like when it came to video cameras?

2. Is there a problem with the basics of chewing gum, chamomile, cauliflower, wine, thyme, oats, ore, or a new one? Is it possible to have a masquerade under the guise of a mouse, a primer, "Oh dear, that does not work for you"?

3. Did the missile manifestation or the missile inversion occur? Are they in the form of an extractor?

4. Do you remember my stories, do you agree with the intentions of your stories? It is not, however, worthwhile to use custom mosaics, which are the mainstay of prevention. You can configure how to completely remove your mice.

Certainly, it is not possible to try your hand at using substandard models. In this case, the result is that the situation is similar to the one we are talking about.

Exercise 13 (Explain Exercise 12)

Explain the need for a situation in which you are dealing with different circumstances.

108

Repair molds, dry cleaning materials and washing machines. By default, you will be able to increase the intensity of the activity and the percentage of activity that you have.

Date	
Subject	
Love	
Mysli	

Try to fill out the form below form:

1. Project management - is it something concrete and objective, or a mix of goals, money, ideas or business? What did it look like when it came to video cameras?

2. Is there a problem with the basics of chewing gum, chamomile, cauliflower, wine, thyme, oats, ore, or a new one? Is it possible to have a masquerade under the guise of a mouse, a primer, "Oh dear, that does not work for you"?
3. Did the missile manifestation or the missile inversion occur? Are they in the form of an extractor?
4. Do you remember my stories, do you agree with the intentions of your stories? It is not, however, worthwhile to use custom mosaics, which are the mainstay of prevention. You can configure how to completely remove your mice.

Certainly, it is not possible to try your hand at using substandard models. In this case, the result is that the situation is similar to the one we are talking about.

Exercise 14

This is a very important moment, and you should take 15-30 minutes to finish the analysis of the two parts. For that which is

109

you should choose the one that you will not find related to your sociophobia.

You need to fill in this request for more than one item at a time. If you want to, you can select any two.

On this and the following page you will need a form for completing this exercise.

If this is not the case, then in the "Workplace" section you will find additional tables.

The main table, which you will find in the following page:

1. Project management - is it something concrete and objective, or a mix of goals, money, ideas or business? What did it look like when it came to video cameras?
2. Is there a problem with the basics, the time, how

much, how much, how much, how much, how much, how much money you have? Is it possible to say "masked under the influence of mysticism", first of all, "it's a joke, it's not a good idea"?

5. Did the missile manifestation or the missile invasion occur? Are they in the form of an extractor?

6. Do you remember my stories, do you agree with the intentions of your stories? It is not, however, worthwhile to use custom mosaics, which are the mainstay of prevention. You can configure how to completely remove your mice.

This is the part where you analyze the contents of your data. The format of the non-modified version will be modified.

Search the form A minimum of three days, in which case there are no more than 10 situations. Get rid of slippery slope 3.6 and get rid of slippery slope slippage.

110

Mosaic analysis: Form A

Date	
Subject	
Love	
Mysli	

Exercise 15

From now on, you will use form B to analyze thoughts instead of form A from exercise 14. This means that after identifying the thoughts that caused the negative experiences, you should spend some time changing those thoughts.

Instructions for the practice of the 14th most

undefeated. Those who need to take 30 minutes to complete the analysis of the microscope and the applications that are from you, the irrational level. In the case of any analysis in which you can express yourself, you can either have any experience for this or that.

This large form will not be able to change. For the implementation of various programs that can be used for analyzing microscopic tools.

Undoubtedly, you will be able to maintain your level of analysis. This will be facilitated, firstly, by your constant practice in performing this exercise, and secondly, the logical errors discussed in section 3.9, common in Secrets of Social phobia.

If you do not have a list of forms for analyzing the microscope, you will need to enter the "Working topics" category.

By filling out the forms on each of the new ones you will find 8 entries

111

1. Do you want to save any of the items you want to buy on a regular basis?
2. In my opinion, how many other things do you find in the best situations?
3. Can I see something on TV, read in a book or magazine, hear on the radio or from other people that would help to prove the veracity of my thought?
4. Can this nibble do not cover the possible effects?
5. Can the other people (can you choose which one specifically) think that, who and what?
6. If this is the case with a lot of people: "Make sure you think about it, if the situation is different"!
7. Are there any other reasons why you and your family are not interested in which specific facts can be

submitted?

8. Can I have the same situation with other types of vehicles that are capable of transporting people? Do you think that this post is not for the faint of heart? (You should be able to use the NEW MUSEUM graph graph.)

If you have any problems with this situation, you can use the "Theoretical books" section of version 3.9.

Mosaic analysis: Form B

Date	
Subject	
Love	
Mysli	
Demonstration missile	
New mice	
Possible natural experiments	

Exercise 16

These are the ones that differentiate the type of logical partitions in previous niche fields. Proven documents that you need on the second page. Each unit can store one of the logical logos.

Find out which ones you can log on to if you want to get rid of the 3.9 "Theoretical book".

Note:
"If you want to get rid of it, it's a waste of time, and you're an idiot, that's an idiot."
This thought assumes that the person will be drawn to the attention of others (2), that they will perceive it negatively (3) and, therefore, they will have a negative opinion about the person as a whole (4).

- If you have a small business, nothing will be of interest to you.
- They are the one who is a pediatrician.
- menus sezachas zasderergaates vec, and K. this is a video.
- The fact that some people are not good at it.
- Roads are not covered.
- mo can not move or drop.
- Well, if anything, it would not work.

I'm at the ebegu, so he doesn't rule.
If you do not have cosmetics, you will not be charged for any of them.

- Nervous, it hurts, like pigs.
- If you want to unlock it, it will not be able to handle it for a long time.
- Mix everything as you like.
- You will not be able to forfeit the money if you make a mistake.
- There are no neurotics, as no one can.
- All things are lawful for me, but I will not be brought under the power of any.
- Well, that's nerve-wracking, as it's not needed by any couple.

8 - 2756
113
Experienced activities in practice 16

- If you have a small business, nothing will be of

interest to you. (2, 3, 4)

- They are the one who is a pediatrician. (2, 3)
- menus sezachas zasderergaates vec, and K. this is a video. (1,2)
- The fact that some people are not good at it. (3, 4, 5)
- Roads are not covered. (2, 3, 4)
- mo can not move or drop. (1)
- Well, if anything, it would not work. (5)

I'm at the ebegu, so he doesn't rule. (1)

If you do not have cosmetics, you will not be charged for any of them. (2, 3, 4)

- Nervous, it hurts, like pigs. (1)
- If you want to unlock it, it will not be able to handle it for a long time. (2, 3, 4)
- Mix everything as you like. (2)
- You will not be able to forfeit the money if you make a mistake. (2, 3)
- There are no neurotics, as no one can. (1, 2, 3, 4.5)
- All things are lawful for me, but I will not be brought under the power of any. (2)
- Well, that's nerve-wracking, as it's not needed by any couple. (2, 3, 4,5)

Interview 17

Please note that some of the new features on this site are supported by regular users.

You can promote your forms of mycelium analysis, which you will find. It is possible that you will need all the primary themes.

Select what is going on in your wallet.

This has been frequently reported. (Listen, what specifically)

114

This is a very interesting tool.

I think the other thing is that it's negative.

I in fact, it would be nice to have a negative note on my account if you are looking for a cell phone or for a new one.
In this case, it is a good idea to add a different size or size to the item.
You can also translate text into text.

Issue 18

If you do not want to miss out on anything you do, it's the result of all the things you've been up to. In the case of a blemish, the most important part is the elimination of this issue.
According to the analysis of all the microscopic forms B in the exercise 14 (you will find in the box office).
By filling out the forms on each of the new ones you will find 8 entries
1. Do you want to find out if any of these are valid on a daily basis? (What did you do with it? How did you find the negative experience?)
2. In my opinion, how many other things do you find in the best situations?
3. Can I see something on TV, read in a book or magazine, hear on the radio or from other people that would help to prove the veracity of my thought?
4. Can this nibble do not cover the possible effects?
5. Can the other people (can they be specific or concrete) think about it, who and what?
8 *
115
6. If this is the case with a lot of people: "Make sure you think about it, if the situation is different"!
7. Are there any other reasons why you and your family are not interested in which specific facts can be submitted?
8. Can I have the same situation with other types of

vehicles that are capable of transporting people? Do you think that this post is not for the faint of heart? (You should be able to use the NEW MUSEUM graph graph.)

Your memory can be used to deliver this cache - this is an idea of your favorite mouse.

Explain these exposures, select options, which you will use in the experimental experiments 19.

Exhibition 19

Provide second-hand experiments. .

In the case of one of the items that need to be listed, you should note that any negative information about what you are doing is valid. You need to be aware of what you are talking about. This file can be used in real time (if you want to scroll). If you use a mirror for this purpose, think about where it is better to put it, or that you will answer the question of why you need it (for example, check if the mascara has not leaked, or check contact lenses, or for a girlfriend - if you are a man). You can also fasten the screen to the toilet and place it in the dark. If you are trying to find the one you are looking for, you should try to find the one you are looking for.

WEEK: from ___

This is the definition of sociophobia in a wide range of specific phenomena (gender, propriety, potency, appraisal, milking and so on).

116

The number of users that you have used is:

The following is the current forecast for VSHGO B:

VOLUME:

General prediction team

all A + all B = all C: ____

Percentage of predicted forecasts (A/S x 100) _______

Additionally, the value of the tag, which my data saves, is ___%.

Exercise 20 (work preparation)

If you find yourself in a different situation, the one you are talking about is the one you are talking about. In fact, the worst thing that can happen is in the middle of nowhere.

Announce the level of the situation you are able to use in your quest.

Explains the experience of the experimenter

Situation	
Volcanic eruption	
Output of your own data	

Proofreading20

For the purpose of filling out the forms with the help of a different type of muesli, the second layer will change your size and

117

that you would like to know more about each other. Depending on the size of the part (possibly, most likely), the number of washes could be reduced.

To fill out the form, each one will have a total of 8 views, which will be added to you as soon as possible.

1. Do you want to find out if any of these are valid on a daily basis? (How many other people did you actually use for this appointment? Please note that it does not work on this one or the other name.
2. In my opinion, how many other things do you find in the best situations? (Is it clear to you that what you are doing is not a good idea?)

3. Can I see something on TV, read in a book or magazine, hear on the radio or from other people that would help to prove the veracity of my thought?
4. Can this nibble do not cover the possible effects?
5. Can the other people (can they be specific or concrete) think about it, who and what?
6. If this is the case with the following words:
7. Are there any other reasons why you and your family are not interested in what concrete facts you can refer to?
8. Can I have the same situation with other types of vehicles that are capable of transporting people? Do you think that this post is not for the faint of heart? (You should be able to use the NEW MUSEUM graph graph.)

Create your own account, you can split your account by selecting the one you want to send to each other.

118

These are the examples, the most popular, the ones that you will find in the experimental experiments 21 - 23.

Exercise 21

Distinguish between us and the ones that take advantage of the fact that there is a lot of people who are interested in it.

Noticeably change something in your clothes (incorrectly fasten buttons, wear something upside down or pull on different socks) or in makeup (draw a pimple on your chin) or change the position of your body (sit emphatically straight, shake your foot, bite your nails). The length of the load is the same as the size of the load. It looks like a niche, which is definitely not one of them.

Increase the percentage of keys that can be used to

make a difference in the amount of time you spend or how much you spend. Remove it from your washing machine.

Your credentials: save size,% value	Daily result: recorded selection,% value:
%	%
%	%

Output:

1. The only thing that makes a difference is that you, as well as you, as a person, you / a person, you are a person.
2. Other fees:

119

Exercise 22

All you have to do is select the number of people you want to share or share in each of them.

It's possible to get rid of it in your flash drive or a dozen of them, and in the end - in college and in winter. If possible, post to select the number of applications you want, the number of which will be displayed next to you.

We recommend that you refrain from asking questions. You could say something like this in response: "I am undergoing a therapeutic course to get rid of my anxiety in society, and...", or "I am worried about my ..."; " Who did you write about?"

• Describe what you are looking for when you start writing for a moment.

• Create, create or share on this note a selection of recent situations. You pay attention to what you are doing, and where you find yourself in the middle of

nowhere.
Sleds to specify one of the most explicit and powerful keys. These will show you cars on the ground. For ethical purposes, slippery forms are used.

Interview 1

(Date: ...) Interview:

120

Interview 2(Date: ...)

Interviews:

Interview 3

(Date: ...) Interview:

Interview 4

(Date: ...) Interview:

Interview 5

(Date: ...) Interview:

121

Interview 6

(Date: ...) Interview:

Interview 7

(Date: ...) Interview:

<u>Exercise 23</u>

You can also specify the correct size of the display to be used for different or different types of applications.
To do this, over the next days or weeks, you should observe someone who exhibits behaviors or features similar to those you fear: redness, nervous tic, trembling, sweating, etc.
When you start to think about a problem with other people, it looks like a bunch of people.
Other capabilities are included in this, allowing you to create your own attempt to find one or another. If you want to try your hand at trying to get rid of it, you should try to get rid of it.

Education 1

________________ Date;

Providence (review)

What is demonstrating?

The right to use a blanket for the removal of this message (review)

____

Education 2

________________ Date

Providence (review)

What is demonstrating?

The right to use a blanket for the removal of this message (review)

____

123

Education 3

________________ Date

Providence (review)

What is demonstrating?

The right to use a blanket for the removal of this message (review)

____

Education 4

________________ Date

Providence (review)

What is demonstrating?

The right to use a blanket for the removal of this message (review)

____

124

Education 5

________________ Date

Providence (review)

What is demonstrating?

The right to use a blanket for the removal of this message (review)

Exercise 24

By doing exercises 21, 22, 23, you can draw your own conclusion about how much others pay attention to the disturbing features of their own behavior or manifestations.

Conclusion: __

Explain the value of the product by the customization of the microsite analysis form.

Exercise 25

The default form of the analysis of the name, the individual form of the name of the one that is the form of the name

125

another, you will forget. Depending on the size of the position of the critical part (possibly, the size of the part), the number of points that can be measured.

1. Do you want to find out if any of these are valid on a daily basis? (How often, according to my observations, did others form a negative opinion in response to my behavior? for example, someone told me directly about it or noticeably changed the attitude towards me.)
2. In my opinion, how many other things do you find in the best situations? (Is it clear to you that in the case of criminals, there is no mention of them?)
3. Can I see something on TV, read in a book or magazine, hear on the radio or from other people that would help to prove the veracity of my thought?
4. Can this nibble do not cover the possible effects?
5. Can other people (you can specify which ones specifically) do you like them?

6. Is it possible to read a lot of people: "Do you think you have a problem, or do you think that the situation is different?"
7. Are there any other reasons why you and your family are not interested in what concrete facts you can refer to?
8. Can I have the same situation with other types of vehicles that are capable of transporting people? Do you think that this post is not for the faint of heart? (You should be able to use the NEW MUSEUM graph graph.)

Submit your request to the subdivision by submitting your submission to the submitter of your subpoena.

Explain this process, use it, and choose it in the experimental experiments 26.

Attention!

Register your data, log in to log logical logs, based on 3.9. If you find yourself in a situation where you have to wait and see what happens next.

126

Exercise 26

As in the game 22, the role of the game is to play a different role. Find out the proper size of the bed, which you can use to cover it. These are options that can be used to deal with issues 22.

You can not just splurge on your favorite things, try out the ones you are looking for, and just go ahead and do them.

As a result, you will find that you have obtained the following information or information about other people and in particular.

Wow, you've got a double whammy, which's a good one. Make sure you have some information on this site, such as what you need to know about it.

If you do not find the one you are looking for, you will be prompted to enter the one you want to send.

Interview 1

(Date: ...)

Interview:

Interview 2

(Date: ...) Interview: _

127

Interview 3

(Date: ...) Interview:

Interview 4

(Date: ...) Interview: _

Exercise 27

When filling out daily thought analysis forms, pay special attention to thoughts that others completely reject you because of one feature of your behavior or appearance. Depending on the size of the position of the critical part (possibly, the size of the part), the number of points that can be measured. It's something you can use to get rid of clutter, and it's hard to get rid of clutter you can handle.

1. Do you want to find out if any of these are valid on a daily basis? (How often, according to my observations, did others form a negative opinion of me as a person, based on the peculiarities of my behavior (appearance)? For example, someone told me directly about it or noticeably changed the attitude towards me.)

128

2. In my opinion, how many other things do you find in the best situations? (Remember, what are the formalities or not of what is the difference between the two, and what are they?)

3. Can I see something on TV, read in a book or magazine, hear on the radio or from other people that would help to prove the veracity of my thought?
4. Can this nibble do not cover the possible effects?
5. Can other people (you can specify which ones specifically) do you like them?
6. Is it possible to read a lot of people: "Do you think you have a problem, or do you think that the situation is different?"
7. Are there any other reasons why you and your family are not interested in what concrete facts you can refer to?
8. Can I have the same situation with other types of vehicles that are capable of transporting people? Do you think that this post is not for the faint of heart? (You should be able to use the NEW MUSEUM graph graph.)

Create your own account, you can split your account by selecting the one you want to send to each other. Explain this process, use the option, which you will use in the experimental experiments 28 and the following.

Attention!

Register your data, log in to log logical logs, based on 3.9. If you find yourself in a situation where you have to wait and see what happens next.

9 - 2756

129

Exercise 28

As in the 22nd and 26th rounds, this game will play a very important role. Look at the different types of solids that are used in the case, and how much of it is used on a given day. You can combine these questions with questions from exercises 22 and 26 You can not only ask them about your features, the manifestation

of which bothers you, but also just talk about different topics.
If you do not know what you are looking for then just leave it at that time. Enhance this message and find it very useful, and concretely about it.
Capture, copy, copy and paste:
• If you want to save money, you can save it to other people who you are and what you are doing.
• How do you get along with someone you care about, and what do you think about me?
Well, you've got a double whammy that keeps you cool. All kinds of items, items, items that you need to buy, even the most expensive ones.
If you do not find the one you are looking for, you will be prompted to enter the one you want to send.
If you find yourself in a situation where you have to pay for other things that you do not know how to do, you can.
Interview 1
(Date: ...)
Interview: __
130
Interview 2
(Date: ...) Interview:
Interview 3
(Date: ...) Interview: _
Interview 4
(Date: ...) Interview: _

Exercise 29

This is one of the great things that we can do to help you get the most out of your data. Alternate attempts to reset or to delete flashbacks by phone. The moment of urgency is the prediction of the names of the people,

as long as it is successful, you will not be able to reach it, but you will not be able to reach it. Provide uncomplicated resources, which you can distribute to different people.
This is the purpose of mini-resizing. The number of dial numbers used by the telephone directory is calculated. Try unsubscribing, downloading, subscribing.
Occupancy scheme (theme - Straightening of roads):
1. Announcement: «We provide a solution for people who use a car. How can I handle unsolicited transactions? »
2. If the answer is yes, ask further: "What would you think if you see a stranger in a store, restaurant or post office and notice that his hands are shaking when he pays for services?".
If you are looking for an unsolicited list of items, please read:
• How are you doing, what do you think is the right thing to do?
• What do you think about the problem?
• What can you do with it?
• Do you think you can do the same thing with the right people?
• Do you remember your note on that item?
This is just one primer. You should ask about the most relevant or unique information that is relevant to you. Create your own unique analytics tool and select current issues for your problem. In this case, you will be able to choose the one that you are looking for, which will be the one you are looking for. Note: "This type of clot, such as complex, neurotic, and so on. p.? ». Upload good results and make sure you remember

them in the video below.
132
*Telephone communication:*1. What is the message?
2. Forecast of results, categories and results
Interview 1
(Date: ...) Interview: _
Interview 2
(Date: ...) Interview: _
133
Interview 3
(Date: ...) Interview:
Interview 4
(Date: ...) Interview: _
Signed out of _____ phone subscribers.
On the occasion of the formation of the menus of the concrete of the concrete subjects / external video: __________

In the case of formatting, the names of the people (or men) in the field of the specific subject (s) /
Tepper, a well-formatted form of analysis of all micelles, emits in the process of production and the sale of such products.
134

<u>Exercise 30</u>

It's certainly not fixed on any negative aspect, we do not want to mention any one. Because you exhibit a certain type of behavior, you may, for example, be afraid that others will consider you neurotic, stupid, fixated, useless or bad person.
Assess the negative results, which will include all the different values that are different from each other.
Distinguish between the different positions of the user, the number of values and the number of entries in each case. 100 - you score and score all the points

absolutely all, 0 - nothing you do not score.
We support the car, the caravan, on the other hand, the best value of the car and the caravan. Distinguish your interest in a 100-ball scale. We name this one, A.
The carpet can be used to cover the floor, the floor, the flooring, the flooring is not covered. Distinguish your interest in a 100-ball scale. We name this group B.
As you can see, the difference between the times and the number of times in the glass window. Support and support, which can also be selected on the basis of a number of other people. "We are strong" - a distinctly challenging category; There are many things to keep in mind. If you want to know where you are going to go, you will find a lot of other people who "do not have a lot of money". Your list can be defined as:

100 Balls	0 Balls
Does not support the time of marriage	Fits in time
Miles / Druze	Simple
Yemeni	Gloomy
Edny	Uninhabited

<u>Table production.</u>

100 Balls	0 Balls
Beautiful / Precious	Ugly
Cylindrical	Slavic
Spooky	Nervous
(Orodishy father/mother)	Ploche
Required partner	i Unreliable
Various drugs	Predator
Good service	Prodigy
Joyful	Patchy house

Tough	Egoist
Uploads of good news	Tumbles only on such interests
The good humor of Emora is unleashed	Does not mention humor
Takes on self-interested ideas	Unknown
General	Molchun
INTERESTED SUBJECT	Hanuda
Animator Listener	Unmanageable
Golden Rocks	Ruki is one of the most popular restaurants
And so on.	And so on.

When it comes to picking up cache, cotyledons, on the other hand, you can play a role for a little or a few ounces.

Appreciate all the quality of your choice. Enter 100, if you want to, that would be another dummies in each case, as you can see. Enter 0, if you prefer, that you otherwise evaluate what is going on in the supported table. If you want to evaluate the selection of the first job you want to send, you will be able to find one. For example, if you think you are the one who is shooting, that out of 100 players each has 10 goals, you must score 10 points each. If you shoot, you will find a dummy, you will lose a lot of money and you will win, you will win 50 points or more.

136

A rating of 0 points indicates that there is another doubt, but in this case there is no doubt that we are nervous.

Shown this, please note that we have two individuals, A. and B., for which we name each other.

List the middle value for each type of property. Select it for both and for two selected individuals.

If you think other people think a particular quality is extremely important, you can double the value of that trait when you summarize the overall score (average). This is a common practice. You will need to sign up for a great deal of cash on hand, which is a great way to get started. This enables us to fixate on the negative aspects of the nature of the eclipse, as well as the difference between. You are trying to find out what we are talking about, that you're trying to name a few things that are important to you, and that you're trying to find them. In this case, you will see two different types of waders in the most realistic sweatshirt, and not just in the black-and-white.

These are the ones that are most important in your situation. 1. It is important to note that the negative value of the value is

the possibility of a possible post / previous video:

2. They support each other as a child, if they choose this subject (in the form of a circle).

3. A) How to evaluate (middle value): _____________

B) Assessment A by name: ________________________

C) Evaluation B. by name: __

4. Other types of characters, on which people draw names, form a different memory and number:

137

Other short characters	Sebie rating	Appraisal A.	Evaluation B.

5. In each case, the number and the number of selected individuals in the 100-point range shall be

different.

6. Select the default value.

7. Remove the slotted middle notes with the theme, the overlays at point 3.

8. Choose a style that you will find in the results of this exercise:

Support the application of other devices (such as the next page).

Supporting the challenge 30

1. It is important to note that the negative value of the subject is possible as well as the following video:

2. If they support me as a child, if I want to share it with you (in the same category):

138

3. A) How to evaluate (middle name): ______________

B) Otsenka A. by name: ________________________

C) Evaluation B. by name: __

4. Other types of characters, on which people draw names, form a different memory and number: ______________

Other short characters	Sebie rating	Appraisal A.	Evaluation B.

5. In each case, the number and the number of selected individuals in the 100-point range shall be different.

6. Select the default value.

7. Remove the slotted middle notes with the theme, the overlays at point 3.

8. Choose a style that you will find in the results of this exercise:

Support the application of custom keys.

Exercise 31

When filling out daily thought analysis forms, pay special attention to thoughts about how terrible it is when others completely reject you or consider you below their level because of one feature of your behavior or appearance. According to the results of the criticisms,

139

those (possibly, mostly with pomegranates), after which all my facts are backed up. It's something you can use to get rid of clutter, and it's hard to get rid of clutter you can handle.

1. Do you want to find out if any of these are valid on a daily basis? (How often, according to my observations, did others form a negative opinion of me as a person, based on one feature of my behavior (appearance)? for example, someone told me directly about it or noticeably changed the attitude towards me.)

9. In my opinion, how many other things do you find in the most favorable situations? (Remember, what are the formalities or not of what is the difference between the two, and what are they?)

2. Can I see something on TV, read in a book or magazine, hear on the radio or from other people that would help to prove the veracity of my thought?

3. Can this nibble do not cover the possible effects?

4. Can the other people (can you choose which one specifically) do you like, who and what?

5. Is it possible to read the following words: "Do you think you are ready to go, or do you think the situation is different"?

6. If this is not the case then maybe your spouse should have an opinion on this topic as well.

7. Can I have the same situation with other types of

vehicles that are capable of transporting people? Do you think that this post is not for the faint of heart? (You will be logged in to the NOW MUSEUM graph).

Submit your request using the submission of your submission to the subpoena, which will allow you to change your submission.

140

Explain what you are doing, select an option, which you will use in the experimental experiment 28 and the following.

Attention!

Register your data, log in to log logical logs, based on 3.9. If you find yourself in a situation where you have to wait and see what happens next.

Exercise 32

This exercise is similar to exercise 30, but in this case it considers the possibility of overly condemning yourself on the basis of any one feature of your behavior or appearance. It's certainly not fixed on any negative aspect, we do not want to mention any one. Because you exhibit a certain type of behavior, you may, for example, be afraid that others will consider you neurotic, stupid, fixated, useless or bad person.

Assess the negative results, which will include all the different values that are different from each other.

Distinguish between the different positions of the user, the number of values and the number of entries in each case. 100 - you score and score all the points absolutely all, 0 - nothing you do not score.

We support the car, the caravan, on the other hand, the best value of the car and the caravan. Distinguish your interest in a 100-ball scale. We name this one, A.

The carpet can be used to cover the floor, the floor, the flooring, the flooring is not covered. Distinguish your interest in a 100-ball scale. We name this group B.

As you can see, there are some things you can do to help me get started. Support and support, as you would.

141

you are always on your phone. "We are strong" - a distinctly challenging category; There are many things to keep in mind. Keep in mind that there are some things that you do not know how to cut down on. Your list can be defined as:

100 Balls	0 Balls
Does not support the time of marriage	Fits in time
Miles / Druze	Simple
Yemeni	Gloomy
Edny	Uninhabited
Beautiful / Precious	Ugly
Cylindrical	Slavic
Spooky	Nervous
(Orodishy father/mother)	Ploche
Required partner	Unauthorized
Various drugs	Predator
Good service	Prodigy
Joyful	Patchy house
Tough	Egoist
Uploads of good news	Tumbles only on such interests
The good humor of Emora is unleashed	Does not mention humor
Takes on self-interested ideas	Unknown
General	Molchun

INTERESTED SUBJECT	Hanuda
Animator Listener	Unmanageable
Golden Rocks	Ruki is one of the most popular restaurants
And so on.	And so on.

When you select the cache, the cadet will be added to your request. Appreciate all the quality of your choice. Paste 100, or your request will be cleared by those who are in the right place at the top of the table. Write 0, if you

142

mummy. with.......... Z........... If you want to evaluate this, you need to create a list, which will show you the type of content. For example, if you think you are out of a total of 100 bullets out of a total of 10 bullets, you will be able to find 10 bullets in the "firefighting" chain. If you choose to play the green and the green, you will find 50 balls for the "blue" cache. A total of 0 balloons can be used for anything in the field, if you shoot them, there is no nerve in the world that we have.

Shown this, please note that we have two individuals, A. and B., for which we name each other.

List the middle value for each type of property. Select it for both and for two selected individuals.

If you want to create a specific type of vehicle, you can specify the value of the item you want to create (if any).

This is a very interesting experience: you will find out what you can do to get the most out of it. This enables us to fixate on the negative aspects of the self-examination of the body, which is also what we are You will find that your credentials are based on the most comprehensive support of all your submissions and queries. This is a chrome-plated, high-waisted, high-waisted, high-waisted, high-waisted, and non-black suede sole.

These are the ones that are most important in your situation.

1. It is important to note that the negative value of the subject is possible as well as the following video:

2. This is the same as the one for the boys (in the second quarter):

143

3. (A) The rate at which the price (average value) is:

B) Otsenka A. by name:

C) Evaluation B. by name:

4. Other short characters, associated with the same:

Other short characters	Sebie rating	Appraisal A.	Evaluation B.

5. In each case, you have to confirm that you have selected the 100-ball scale, that is to say that you are one of them.

6. Select the default value.

7. Remove the slotted middle notes with the theme, the overlays at point 3.

8. Find outings, which are based on the results of this event:

Please note that there is an issue with other countries.

144

<u>Proofreading</u>33

Check out 29 and provide a comprehensive phone call. Accentuate the words, which are not related to each of the following points:

• Do you choose the best cocoa-like scoop that has the specificity of a specific negative one?
• What kind of service can be used (the use of such keys, splits, etc.)?
Telephone communication:
3. What is the message?
4. Forecast forecast, category and category:
Interview 1
(Date: ...) Interview: _
10 - 2756
145
Interview 2
(Date: ...) Interview: _
Interview 3
(Date: ...) Interview: _
Interview 4
(Date: ...) Interview: _
Signed out of _____ phone subscribers.
Tepper, a well-formatted form of analysis of all micelles, emits in the process of production and the sale of such products.
146

Exercise 34

Keep a "Positive Journal" in which for 5-10 minutes daily you will write down what positive things happened to you during the day or what positive qualities you possess.
Each day you can get all the quotes from the previous day. Please note that you can delete all compliments.
In this "Rabotechi tetradi" you need 14 forms. It is recommended to have a minimum of 14 times, another level, on the basis of two points. For example, if you are interested in it, you can have a good practice, which will be the most successful of them all.

Positive Dnieven
Date: ______________________________
Positive Trade / Custody
Date: ____________________________
Positive Trade / Custody
Date: ____________________________
Positive Trade / Custody
S * 147
Date: ____________________________
Positive Trade / Custody
Date: ____________________________
Positive Trade / Custody
Date: ____________________________
Positive Trade / Custody
Date: ____________________________
Positive Trade / Custody
Date: ____________________________
Positive Trade / Custody
148
Date: ____________________________
Positive Trade / Custody
Date: ____________________________
Positive Trade / Custody
Date: ____________________________
Positive Trade / Custody
Date: ________________________
Positive Trade / Custody
Date: ____________________________
Positive Trade / Custody
149
Date: ________________________
Positive Trade / Custody

Interview 35

Create a list of names that you will find that are

positive about you. Apply to those who are most interested in you.

What positive do you think we are?

Date: ______________________ Comments:

Date: ______________________ Comments:

Date: ______________________ Comments:

Date: ______________________ Comments:

Date: ______________________ Comments:

150

Date: ______________________ Comments:

Date: ______________________ Comments:

Exercise 36

It may be one or two phrases, including all the facts, that you MUST use as a whole. There are only two positive reviews.

Note:

"I am an honest and kind man"

"I think the only ones"

"I'm proud of you and my mother-in-law"

"I have a lot of polite users"

Write down the phrases on the card. If you want to get rid of this badge, you should try to get rid of it and get some news out of the way.

Positive results:

151

Proofreading37 *

Notice of the time required, listed on the cassette. Do not overdo it with good food. This is an unsolicited application, as is the case with the following. Do not overdo it with the sledgehammer. The most successful applications do not have enough time to spare. Make sure you keep track of the issues. Here are some suggestions on how to look or get an appointment for antique items. Anything that has been given a good

deal of support in trying this option may have been completed by one or more.
Date, entry to, entry post, entry
Date, entry to, entry post, entry
Date, entry to, entry post, entry
Date, entry to, entry post, entry
* If you have the ability to create a cassette or a compact disc that contains the text you want to produce.
152
Date, entry to, entry post, entry
Date, entry to, entry post, entry
Date, entry to, entry post, entry
Date, entry to, entry post, entry
Date, entry to, entry post, entry
Date, entry to, entry post, entry

Exercise 38

These can be used to fill out a series of recordings, recorded on cassette tapes. It is located on the B.
153
Anything that has been successfully resolved to support this challenge may be deprecated by one or more.
Date, entry to, entry post, entry
Date, entry to, entry post, entry
Date, entry to, entry post, entry
Date, entry to, entry post, entry
Date, entry to, entry post, entry
Date, entry to, entry post, entry
Date, entry to, entry post, entry
154
Date, entry to, entry post, entry
Date, entry to, entry post, entry
Date, entry to, entry post, entry

Exercise 39

You can start exercise 3. Once you have managed to relax with this exercise, you can proceed to perform the next, but not earlier than 10 times the repetition of this exercise.

Date, entry to, entry post, entry
Date, entry to, entry post, entry
Date, entry to, entry post, entry
155
Date, entry to, entry post, entry
Date, entry to, entry post, entry
Date, entry to, entry post, entry
Date, entry to, entry post, entry
Date, entry to, entry post, entry
Date, entry to, entry post, entry
Date, entry to, entry post, entry

Interview 40

You can support this application by following this example, which is a short one. Do not override the default attempt to your device, do not try to get rid of it properly. This entry is for a minimum of 20 rs.

Date, entry to, entry post, entry
Date, entry to, entry post, entry
Date, entry to, entry post, entry
Date, entry to, entry post, entry
Date, entry to, entry post, entry
Date, entry to, entry post, entry
157
Date, entry to, entry post, entry
Date, entry to, entry post, entry
Date, entry to, entry post, entry
Date, entry to, entry post, entry
Date, entry to, entry post, entry

Exercise 41

Complete the fourth request without cassettes. The average size of a range is from 1 to 10. You will find relaxation rates for relaxation. Remember to use the "RACE" button. Do not specify the extension of this option, except for the default settings.

Date, entry to, entry post, entry

158

Date, entry to, entry post, entry

Date, entry to, entry post, entry

Date, entry to, entry post, entry

Date, entry to, entry post, entry

Date, entry to, entry post, entry

Date, entry to, entry post, entry

Date, entry to, entry post, entry

Date, entry to, entry post, entry

Date, entry to, entry post, entry

Date, entry to, entry post, entry

Exercise 42

Complete application for the same number of objects as follows:

STOUSE

Date, entry to, entry post, entry

Date, entry to, entry post, entry

Date, entry to, entry post, entry

Date, entry to, entry post, entry

160

Date, entry to, entry post, entry

2. FRIENDLY

Date, entry to, entry post, entry

Date, entry to, entry post, entry

Date, entry to, entry post, entry

Date, entry to, entry post, entry

Date, entry to, entry post, entry

3. PRIDE VACCANUM RADIO

Date, entry to, entry post, entry
11—2756
161
Date, entry to, entry post, entry
Date, entry to, entry post, entry
Date, entry to, entry post, entry
Date, entry to, entry post, entry
4. PRIZE VAKNONOM TV
Date, entry to, entry post, entry
Date, entry to, entry post, entry
Date, entry to, entry post, entry
162
Date, entry to, entry post, entry
Date, entry to, entry post, entry
5. WHERE DOES THE PRINCIPAL PAYMENT
Date, entry to, entry post, entry
Date, entry to, entry post, entry
Date, entry to, entry post, entry
Date, entry to, entry post, entry
Date, entry to, entry post, entry
and *
163
6. WHERE'S THE WORLD OF STONE
Date, entry to, entry post, entry
Date, entry to, entry post, entry
Date, entry to, entry post, entry
Date, entry to, entry post, entry
Date, entry to, entry post, entry
7. (PLEASE REMEMBER THE SAME)
Date, entry to, entry post, entry
Date, entry to, entry post, entry
164
Date, entry to, entry post, entry
Date, entry to, entry post, entry

Date, entry to, entry post, entry

Exercise 43

Expose the background of a circle in an empty hole and place a comma-nib in a glass. Refer to the name of your post and the title of the post. Some may be able to display the page, but you will not be able to preview it.

Do not overwrite an application on a full table, you can configure any entries and delete any entries. Note:

How are you doing? Hello. The menu ... (present) Select to enter. F does not present this. However, the book has not been updated yet. How much money do you spend on cinema tickets? I domuma, kak milo s vashastey steruni priglacite menu. If it's a deal, it's a hot topic, I'm not a big fan of drugs. • Do you want to get rid of it properly, do not try it?

It is recommended that you do not have a 5 star rating. If you have an issue with this article, please leave a comment below.

165

Explains how to complete worksheets:

Date: _ Notes:

Date: _ Notes:

Date: _ Notes:

Date: _ Notes:

Date: _ Notes:

Exercise 44

In the case of slippery slopes, you should practice cleaning on contact. For this purpose, there is an unusual amount of glass in the glass, which is used in small or medium-sized windows. If you are trying to delete a message from a user,

166

try to find a second sequel. It may not be possible to

display unsolicited data, but it is not possible to create a password that can be used to display the device. The total load is not 10 rms. Each file will be checked.
Explains the requirements for contact glazing:
Date: _ Notes:
Date: _ Notes:
Date: _ Notes:
Date: _ Notes:
Date: _ Notes:
167

Exercise 45

Log in to your phone's recorder. For this cell, use the display 43 of the frame, which can be mounted on a recorder. Listen to files and correct the defects that the user is looking at. Remember that your goals do not go down well with you.

Examination of the distribution of relevant languages:

Volume: __
:Accuracy: __
Network speed:
____
Intonations:
____
Other Characteristics:
____

Exercise 46

Attach to the recorder shortcut to your phone and listen to it. Create an account, which can be used as a result of your race, cast the ballot box, and the cost of the match.

Create your own account, which you will find on your account, and create your own accounts. Support the casting of 3 razors.

Explains how to debug your passwords:

168

Date:

Category: __________

Number: __

Network speed: _______

Intonations: _________

Other features:

Date: _______________

Category: __________

Number: __

Network speed: _______

Intonations: _________

Other features:

Date: _______________

Category: __________

Number: __

Network speed: _______

Intonations: _________

Other features:

169

Exercise 47

In the case of postal data, it is recommended that you keep a close eye on other types of data. You can delete this and that in the first place, but you can only use the same size as you would like to use. The following notifications (not all) can be shared, broadcasting television programs. Send messages (ideally - if you do not have one) separate your outputs on each aspect, which are selected in the context. It is recommended that you do not have a 6 time rating. If there is a possibility, we will point out the meaning of what we are talking about (memory or speed).

Announcement of the new post of other people:
Date: -
City: _____
Who: _______
Here is one:
Glass contact:
Phone number:
Click on the link:
Range style: ___
Conclusion: _________
170
Date:
City: ________
Where: __________
This is the date: ___
Glaze contact: Phone location: Line selection:
Range style: ___
Conclusion: _________
Date:
____
City: ____
To:
____
___
This is one of them:
____
Glass contact:
____
Phone number: ____________________________
b_________
Excerpt from:
____
Theme type:
____

171
Output:
Date: _ City: Who:
Here is one:
Glass contact: Phone location: _ Line selection:
Range style: ___
Conclusion: ________
Date:
City: Which:
Here is one:
Glazing Contact: Phone Number: Line Size: Range Type: ___
172
Output:
Date: __________
City: ________
Where: __________
This is the date: ___
Glaze contact: Phone location: Line selection:
Range style: ___
Conclusion: _________

Exercise 48

If you do not have a video recorder and you do not have the option to copy it, it can be used for this purpose.

Remove from the camcorder anytime you need it or try to find and listen to it. Please note that you may have access to all your submissions. Prompt your memory to be able to record and display your memory. Select all items in your account.

This request does not have a limit of 3 times.

Check out how to monitor video logging:

173

Date:

Glass contact: __
Phone number: __
Click here: __
Range style: _____
Other notes:
Date: ____________
Glass contact: __
Phone number: __
Click here: __
Range style: _____
Other notes:
Date: ____________
Glass contact: __
Phone number: __
Click here: __
Range style: _____
Other notes:

VHIBI
Exhibition 49

Please note and review all non-negotiable items in your list, such as those in this category. The size of the case should be defined as new, new and paid in special formats. This entry is for a term not 10 times.

If possible, try a new level, which is within our range (remember or change), select your bet.

Post new posts:

Date: _ City: City:
Here are the details:
Glass contact:
Phone number:
Excerpt from: _____________
Theme type: ________________
Results and plan for the next race:

175
Date: __
City: By:
Here are the details:
Glass contact:
Phone number:
Excerpt from the link: Range of men: ___
Results and plan for the next race:
Date:
City: By:
Here are the details:
Glazing Contact: Phone Number: Line Size: Range Type: ___
176
Results and plan for the next race:
Date: _
City:
With which:
Here are the details:
Glass contact:
Phone number:
Excerpt from the link: Range of men: ___
Results and plan for the next race:
Date:
City:
With which:
Here are the details:
Glass contact:
Phone number:
12 - 2756
177
Excerpt from: _______________
Theme type: __________________
Results and plan for the next race:

Exercise 50

Create a list of entries, which will be used in nebulae. Suggest all situations, in which it is possible to have a message: if there is a transport, you will be able to do this. d. Try your best, possibly, and offer better variants of situations.

Your passwords:

Situation 1:

____

1. 2. 3. 4. 5.

Situation 2:

____

1. 2. 3. 4. 5.

Situation 3:

____

1. 2. 3. 4. 5.

Exercise 51

Distribute unsolicited and unsolicited proclamations.

If you want to close the window, you will need to change it as well.

What do you think about it? Written / closed

What do you expect from a popular pipe? Written / closed

How to work? Written / closed

Do not you understand whether it is white or not? Written / closed

Everything on the porch? Written / closed

Do you work in an insurance company? Written / closed

What a beautiful dove, do you think? Written / closed

The most common types of items you need are new.

Proven remarks in Exercise 51:

What do you think about it? Written

What do you expect from a popular pipe? Lacquered. Excerpts: What kind of pipe do you like? How to work? Written

Do not you understand whether it is white or not? Lacquered. Excerpts: How did you find the right recovery? Everything on the porch? Lacquered. How to deal? Do you work in an insurance company? Lacquered. Would you like to date a friend?

What a beautiful dove, do you think? Lacquered. Explained: What do you think about it?

12 *

179

Exercise 52

You can quickly build and print hidden and sacred objects. In fact, it is not possible for them to monitor television programs in which people live. If you are looking for a predetermined or unreported prompt, enter it in the graph of this topic.

Descendants and hidden motions, television projections

Date	Written	Lacquered

Proofreading53

Read for yourself what you need to know when you are ready for all kinds of bad things. You can find what you are looking for. It is possible to use this information on other types of equipment, such as those you do not want to use. It is recommended that you do not have a 5 star rating.

Explains the fulfillment of the requirements of the proclamation:

180

Date: _____

Remarks:

Date: _____

Remarks:

Date: _____

Remarks:

Date: _____

Remarks:

Date: _____

Remarks:

Exercise 54

Work on any of the key issues that may arise, such as your partner, your partner or your partner.

In each case, your attempt will expose you to something that you did not want to delete, and you will find out what you are looking for. In each case, the following data is summarized in your subpoena and subpoena.

181

This request does not appear to be 5 times for each one you want to send.

Problems solving your request:

Date: ____________________________

Declared / closed entries:

Reports:

Compliments:

Logo:

Remarks:

Date: ____________________________

Declared / closed entries:

182
Reports:
Compliments:
Logo:
Remarks:
Date: ____________________________
Declared / closed entries:
Reports:
Compliments:
Logo:
Remarks:
183
Date:
Declared / closed entries:
Reports:
Compliments:
Logo:
Remarks:
Date: ____________________________
Declared / closed entries:
Reports:
Compliments:
184
Logo:
Remarks:

Exercise 55

In fact, there are many things that can be done to help you get started. Keep up the good content and make sure you have a good look at the ones you are looking for. Submit specific queries to select the value of the relevant key. It is generally possible to divide the number of characters by the number of characters.

List of companies to listen to the following:

Date: _

Declared / closed entries:
Reports:
Compliments:
185
Logo:
Remarks:
Date: ________________________
Declared / closed entries:
Reports:
Compliments:
Logo:
Remarks: ___
Date: ________________________
Declared / closed entries:
186
Reports:
Compliments:

____

Total: __
:Notes: __

Exercise 56

Provides the best known phrase, which you can use in different situations.

The most common phrases:
Situation 1:
187
Situation 2:
Situation 3:
Situation 4:
Situation 5:
Situation 6:

Proofreading57

In the case of unscrupulous data on the case, you should try to save the property. Define how well these

techniques work for you and your loved ones. Delete what is known, the crane more than one note, the procedure does not show a smooth flow. All for the same level - choose the best new ones.
188
Maintenance Challenge:
Date: ___________________
If you want to save the message:
How to save a message:
Remarks:
Date: ___________________
If you want to save the message:
_How to save a message:
Remarks:
Date: ___________________
If you want to save the message:
189
How to save a message:
Remarks:

Exercise 58

New premiums are offered. Please tell, whats the story of them big puppys ..... If not, select and delete scripts. Regular items are listed on the second page.
1. Your customer will provide us with information.
2. On the other hand, you have to deal with the good news.
3.M-m-m-m ...

Real estate activities 58

*Your customer will provide us with information.*This is the best way to write a personal statement: "I Am Duma, that is what you are actually referring to.
This is a good thing that you can easily get rid of.
It is very clear that it is concrete and has a good shape, as in the positive aspect, it is "I think it's something I'm

doing.

M-m-m-m ...

Very specific concrete: "It is not possible to pre-empt this large-scale sauce, as it were. I'm domuma, on horscheh podhodite k g goyadine."

Proofreading59

These are the main products of the same design compliments. Add a compliment to your request

190

I do not understand the meaning of the words. They do not need to be registered with the same-level vehicle. You can practice practicing with your lightning bolts or drums. Obviously this is not a bad thing at all. It is used in the practice of small-scale, collegiate and t. d.

Do not overdo it with these ointments, as well as the extracts and creams of this kind of effect. It is possible to use it to record many videos of compliments, which we will share with you.

/. Delete comma-nibud compliment on the interior of this home. It's not really a bad race. Note:

•This is what you call a beautiful divan, a cross, a chair and so on. d.

I think that ... very hoshsho comes with ...

• This is ... very beautiful, like a watch.

• I love this fantasy film.

2. Divide the comma-nibud compliment by the tag that is on the set. It's not really a bad race. Note:

•It's good, but it's just what's special.

• I'm in fact, you will always need a new one.

• I domuma, u uysten chisto cubrale zes.

• I really like to mess with you.

• A mile away from your pages, which you will find. I'm a day-it is certainly the price.

3. Distribute a comma-nibud compliment to a particular person. It's not really a bad race. Note:

- I domuma, what u are obviously prequel.
- I in this case, what you are looking for is a glass slide.
- I Duma, it's a bicycle, what do you think is so beautiful-

the last day of the week.

4. Distribute a comma-nibud compliment to a group of distinguished customers or recipients. It's not really a bad race. Note:

- This is what you need.

191

- I Like, you have an accurate key.
- You are on the right track. I think it's weird.

5. Separate comma-nibud compliment, which you will like. This is not a very popular article.

Complimentation training test:

Date: _______

Compliment:

Response: ____

Remarks: __

Date: _______

Compliment:

Response: ____

Remarks: __

Date: _______

Compliment:

192

Response:

:Notes: __

Date: __________________

Compliment:

____

Response:

____

:Notes: __

Date: __________________

Compliment:

____

Response:

____

:Notes: __

Exercise 60

The most common of these is the primer of reaction to compliments. Distinguish, support them for the first models, described in "Theoretical books". Do not delete, delete files and delete yourself. Regular sales of items on the second page.

1. *Compliment:*"I think, this is a very important project." Response: "I received the recipe from Mary".
13 - 2756 193

2. *Compliment:*"You're fast-forwarded to work." This menu is intended to be a unique feature ». Response: "I just finished working".

3. *Compliment: "/*hey, you wash new ones that are obvious to you ». Response: "I have a lot of nice lenses, but I'll be able to persuade you."

Exercise information on practice 60

1. *Preferred reaction:*«Thanks. This was done in the same part of the race. I'm getting a recipe from Mary ».

(Preferred variant: print a compliment, remove a substantial coin.)

2. *Preferred reaction:*"That's a mile, that's what you're talking about. I'm seriously working on the team."

(Preferred variant: print a compliment, remove a substantial coin.)

3. *Preferred reaction:*"How nice, it's what you're talking about." Well, at least I did not go down without explaining myself first.

(Preferred variant: print a compliment, remove a substantial coin.)

Exercise 61

In the case of secondary needles, your reaction to a compliment is based on the case models. You can specify which one to use.

It's possible that you will not be able to reach the end of your life or that you will be rewarded with a compliment.

Complimentation reaction to compliment

Date: _______

Compliment:

Response: ____

Remarks:

Date: _______

Compliment:

Response: ____

Remarks:

Date: _______

Compliment:

Response: ____

Remarks:

n *

195

Exercise 62

The new prime minister is not known. Please tell, whats the story of them big puppys ..... Do not delete, delete files and delete yourself.

1. It is possible that you can use it for the purpose of using a simple home page.
2. Do not override the subject, which will be your

home page and will display the TV, as well as the amount of work you have done. All items must be checked. It may be a cigarette smoke propeller. We do not want to tell you all about what you want, do not you?

Bros., you are the best friend!

Real estate deals 62

Testing in the models with models:

/. "If you have a hotel, you can book and try to find me." This is the fold of the slippery slope. Do you remember me? » (Proofreading: create from your own name, do not translate a dictionary, create a name and a specific one.)

2. «If you have a home screen and watch the TV. Good? »(Proofreading: does not include, is concrete and concrete, does not have a different meaning, does not show different colors).

3. "I However, those who prefer to enjoy your nose in my della. Good? »(Proofreading: score from your own name, name and specifics, play another game).

Exercise 63

You will be able to see the results of your visit. Please find any type of sample that you have in common with other people. It may be possible to talk to someone else or

196

lightning fast - it's a very good one. It is possible to practice this practice with my favorite characters, colleges and so on. d.

The following pages will show you how to create and manage your own page. Use these forms and to record important videos, which you can choose from.

In the next step, you should try to find the "ideal" design.

To make sure that you finish your shots in the video. If you do not have time for writing a post, please submit a post, as well as any questions or comments you may have.

1. Do not talk to someone on the phone but do not listen to them. Note:

• If you want to go out of your way, you will find out more ...

• If you have a hotel where you can send an information-

About ... Are you working on it?

• x Hotel bye, you are here for my menu. I've been warned

spout of nectar, which you can pick up. Good?

• I want to present you a movie at the cinema in this movie. What?

2. Serve this libo in a coffee shop or restaurant for many more people.

Note:

• I use mineral water with lemonade.

• x hotel with other selfies; it is very gray.

• The hotel has plenty of room to spare.

Can't you guess what is in the kitchen?

• I though you try to add a lot of water to my na-
pitok.

3. Try to get something done. This request does not appear to be a true race.

• x hotels near you in this book. Are not you a protégé?

• I would like to give you 10/20/50 dollars.

Which name is this?

I x would like you to help me... i You deal with it?

197

4. Do not overdo it. This request does not appear to be

a true race.
Note:
I what are you trying to do without deleting ... Good?
• If you do not find yourself in a predicament, you may find yourself in a predicament.
meni. Good?
5. Offer a chemo-friendly key. This request does not appear to be a true race.
Note:
• I hotel to project in case of loss to me, which is a ban-
with a theme, the title page and the title. Aren't you a protégé?
• If you want to send something to someone, please .... No
can I tell you what I can do?
• There are plenty of things that you can watch on TV. Can't you agree?
6. Assemble the unit cleanly. Failure to execute calls will not occur.

Provision for "ideal" design

Date: ________________
View (close window):
Specify specific points for project design:
Date: ________________
View (close window):
Specify specific points for project design:
Date: ________________
View (close window):
Specify specific points for project design:
Date: ________________
View (close window):

Determine specific points according to the projection

of the sample

Date: ________________

View (close window):

Specify specific points for project design:

Exercise 64

Newly viewed primaries are displayed on the screen. Please tell, whats the story of them big puppys ..... Do not delete, delete files and delete yourself.

1. There is no such thing as self-promotion for cars.
2. Do not try to get rid of them on your phone. There are also many types of products, and you can choose the one that is best for you, and not the best. And this is because foam does not work on nerves.

I do not think that we have a very good reputation. Undoubtedly, this is not a very good idea - to take a drug with a drug for a long time. It is possible, however, that we do not know how to store it and we are able to deplete another drug on nerves.

200

Common objects in practice 64

1. There is no such thing as a motorcycle with you. I do not like guns. You can get rid of clutter you need.(Speech: reading, contraption.)

2. Sm. p. 1.(Proofreading: speed, not sloppy, not very easy to use.)

3. No, it's not trying to get rid of you. . I do not think that we're doing anything else that is sufficient. Can't you find the best news yet?(Translations: name, isolated from your subject, only one entry, counter-presentation, not an independent dictionary.)

Exercise 65

All you have to do is choose the right one. Find any type of sample that you want to buy. You can practice practicing with your favorite drug or with light bulbs.

Obviously this is a very nice bed. It will be possible for you to complete an exercise with a variety of comics, colleges and so on. d.

The following pages will show you how to create and manage your own page. You can use these forms to record other videos, which you can choose from.

In the next step, you should try to find the "ideal" design for the test.

To make sure that you get rid of clutter you need on the video screen. If you do not have time for writing a post, please submit a post, as well as any questions or comments you may have.

Do not forget that you can try to save the name on the topic and quickly submit it to the polling station. Any time you choose to try, remember what you are looking for and what effect it will have.

201

*1. Select the desired size of the blanket. This request does not appear to be a true race. (If you are in the wrong position to submit this application, please refer to the practitioner.)*Note:

• It is not possible to present this one as a whole. This is what will happen. Good?

• NO. What are we talking about and what are we not talking about?

• NO. I'm not a bitch. I want to share with your position.

• Not, it does. I definitely like everything I do. St is stretched out with chem. Can I make it a store?

*2. Excerpt from the application (does not mean trash).*Note:

• There is no such thing as a picture. There is no such thing as a scooter. Can you have a better time in the theater?

• I do not remember the date of the coffee. It is possible to bite, save-
or?

• There is no way to get rid of these losses. This club may have a very good reputation, but it's all there is to it.

*3. Exclude from shared offerings. This request does not appear to be a true race (possibly, by phone).*Note:

• There is no warning for this. Do you recommend this?

• If you choose to play, you will not receive any pro-blemishes.

• There is no such thing as a full-fledged post. This is just a sign of the times.

• It can not be undone. I really like it. Do you want to deal with this premium?

*4. Find out the most important person in social situations. Do not try to change the menu.*Note:

• It is not able to provide you first. I really like it.

• No, thank you. (Who is posting on mailings.)

• Not, it's mostly expensive.

202

5.

*Be on the lookout for comedy-nibudi sami. This request does not appear to be valid.*Replace forms on adjacent pages.

Examination at the end of the exam

Date: _________________

Rating (close range):

Basic positions in the selection process:

Examination at the end of the exam

Date: _________________

Rating (register):

Basic positions in the selection process:

Examination at the end of the exam

Date:

Rating (close range):

Basic positions in the selection process:

Examination at the end of the exam

Date: ________________

Rating (close range):

Basic positions in the selection process:

Examination at the end of the exam

Date: ________________

Rating (close range):

Basic positions in the selection process:

Exercise 66

It is not uncommon for us to have primary reassessment at the outlet. Please tell, whats the story of them big puppys ..... Do not delete, delete files and delete yourself.

/. Rating: "No, it can not help you. I will only be entered in the default area. " Response: "If you have a problem, you will die."

2. *Rating:*"It is not possible to estimate the number of projects." Response: "Do you have a prediction, what problem do you have?"

3. *Rating:*"No, it's not a post. It is not possible to support such a serious compromise ». Response: "Good, get it".

Common objects in practice 66

1. *«Very Hall. It is not known that you are silently dying. Can you find out what you need in the case of menus? »*(Excerpt: scan your cubs, preview your polls, select alternate preambles).

2. *"It's well developed, but it's not worth it. There is a*

lot of hard work that can be done by anyone. Can it be, if you want to know, what can I do for you? »(Excerpts: find what you are looking for in your book, first review, alternate offerings.)

3. «It is not possible to estimate what it is. Now it seems that what you are trying to do is not work for you. "(Excerpt: Explain what you see on your pages, see the nickname of the polls.)

Exercise 67

In fact, there are a number of cases where the practice is based on the number of cases in which the model is based. All files must be registered.

205

To make sure that you do not have a partner or a role-playing game, just ask them.

Problems responding to the issue in the process of being executed

Date: ____

Where to go and where: ________________________

My Response to Rating: _____________________

:Notes: __

Problems responding to the issue in the process of being executed

Date: ________________

Where to go and where: __

My reaction to the review:

:Amechania: _____

206

Problems responding to the issue in the process of being executed

Date: ______________

Where to go and where:

My reaction to the review:

Remarks:

Exercise 68

Newly reviewed primary reviews. Please tell, whats the story of them big puppys ..... Do not delete, delete files and delete yourself.

It is customary to monitor slides on slides.

1. It is not possible for you to remember the options you want when you enter your password?
2. Stop using. You will not be able to access nickel files. You save and treat each other with a lot of money.
3. What a joy!

Common objects in practice 68

1. "If you want to get rid of it, you will need to get rid of it." The fabric of the washcloth and the purse are applied to each of them. If you want to get rid of clutter you may need, you will be able to select the ones you are looking for and not the ones you want to play. Good? » (Excerpts: from such names, both concrete and concrete, not a slavish one.)

207

2. "I want to delete your new pages. I will always be able to reach you. Why are we not trying to get rid of some strange things, first of all, or more? What do you think about it? (Proofreading: Critique every single position, name and specific, alternate prediction, percussion definition).
3. "I smell a terrible smell from you. Let us give you a chair, and let us give you a shower and a drink. Aren't you a protégé? » (Proofreading: from your name, alternate preamble, realignment and realignment.)

Exercise 69

You will be able to review critical reviews of the topic. This type of critical compilation allows you to create different types of files. You can use the paint to wash or dry the paint - it is very easy to use. You will be able to practice this practice with a wide range of people, colleges and so on. d.

The following pages are filled out, formatted, as well as some of the criticisms and all of them. Possibly you can use these pages to list other critical videos that we cover. The most important thing you can do is criticize the "ideal" topic.

To support and critique any critical developments that may have occurred. If you are not into this type of business, you will need the following, as well as any information or suggestions that may be useful to you.

/. Criticism of the interior of the house in the guest house. This request does not appear to be a true race.

Note:

• I do not think that this cover is a good one for a divan.

It is best to look at other areas.

• Your home will be inaccurate. Can I help you get rid of it?

208

2. Criticism of those who love religion. This request does not appear to be a true race.

Note:

• I Duma, what is definitely going on - to give you three hours ago. I do not live in cafes in the unit. Are you awake, what do you think about slides?

• I Subscribe to this post as many links as possible. This concludes that it is worth noting that many have been tested. In fact, the slides in the slide are very small. Good?

• You are the one who is not the one who made it. I'm sure enough to sniff. Can this be a fast and easy way to get started?

3. Criticism of the characteristics of drug addicts. This

request does not appear to be a true race.

Note:

• I in fact, there are some things that you can do. The same thing

will perform.

I in fact, there is always a costume in a restaurant. You are not

what fast bistro do you recommend?

• If you want to change the display. You can not

do you have a fair amount of groceries?

• By default, these messages do not appear on your screen.

4. Explain the criticisms that you may have received in private. This request does not appear to be valid.

Criticism of the topic of critique

Date: ____________________

Criticism (Listed Zone):

14 - 2756

209

Critical moments in the critique:

Date: ____________________

Criticism (Listed Zone):

Critical moments in the critique:

Date: ____________________

Criticism (Listed Zone):

Critical moments in the critique:

Date: ____________________

Criticism (Listed Zone):

Critical moments in the critique:

Exercise 70

The most notoriously primitive reactions to criticism. Please tell, whats the story of them big puppys ..... Do not delete, delete files and delete yourself.

/. Criticism: "Oh, I'm sorry, there's a lot of bad guys in

this post. It's good that I'm proud of having a lot of fun. X However, what you are talking about is a consumer. Good? » Response: "Yes, it's steel and steel is a bit fast, but it's all possible."

2. Criticism:"I'm sorry, you've been isolated and have no deal for other people. I recommend that you manage the name of the project ». Response: "What are you talking about?"

Real estate deals 70

1. "I feel terrible. What do you think, what do you do when you have a lot of mistakes? I am proud of you. I'm sure this is a bad thing for me, but I've really needed a quick fix. I have a lot of ideas in the budget, but I have a lot of ideas about how to do it. (Implementation: summing up, summarizing.)

2. «I am very old. What do you really understand, what are you talking about? At the same time, it is a good idea to try another game. There is currently no such thing as a search engine. I need to graduate with an exam ». (Excerpts: the number of cues, summaries, quizzes, and the number of conspiracies mentioned above).

Exercise 71

On the other hand, it is necessary to focus on the model of critique behavior. All files are registered

14 *

211

t, as is the case. At the very least you can try your best to play the role of a critic or whatever you want to reach.

Real Estate Release of Criticism

Date:

What is critical:

My reaction to the criticism:

Remarks:

Proofreading72

Distribute as many cards as you want from the detailed description. Buy a package of books for collection (size 5x3 or 13x8 cm).

For each card of the most common type of application.

Depending on the size of the problem, the numbers are 0 to 100, and the current level is very high.

Manage clutter, as well as clutter clutter. Some of them may not be able to complete the Kaki-Libo challenge, which you will need to follow. You have selected the following names. Delete as many large cards as possible.

212

Find out what you can do with issues 4 and 5, where you will find situations, results in this and that type.

You need to fill out the name of the game you want on the cards. Create your own memory support on this site.

Please note that each and every one of you will be asked about all the cards that your sociophobia will use.

Proofreading73

This is the moment when you need to create a plan, place it, and go to the next level. On the other hand, it is possible to send a ball to the luminaries of the level of the new ones, according to the number of cards in the final year.

You do not specify the range, the range you want to use, and the range you want to use is different.

Planned space even though there is no need to add any details. You can plan as many, as well as unique balloons, which can be found in the drawing of needles. If you are streamed in the same way as the one you are looking for, you will be prompted by the default prompt. If you plan to redesign new posters, each strategy will have a different set of options for each item.

A series of scores that can be found in the results of the search results

Needle ______________________________

Needle ______________________________

Needle ______________________________

213

Needle ______________________________

Needle ______________________________

Needle ______________________________

Needle ______________________________

Needle ______________________________

Needle ______________________________

Needle ______________________________

Exercise 74

You will be able to follow the completion of the download process. Before you start an exercise from any card, write down what you are going to do and what degree of tension you assign to performing this exercise (see next page).

Proanalize your mouse, display the tree, and change it as well, as in level 5. It is possible that they are yours. In order to fulfill the requirements, new mice are added.

Support even the most important social novels play a role in this exercise and follow-up. If you choose to do so, you can support and support the application in the process of execution and / or the application. You can select the type of application you want. If you want to complete an exercise, you must present yourself as well.

Post an application request, as well as any request and any requests you may have.

Prove the application to your wallet, since the application does not support the default level. This is related to the personal bestsellers, as well as the high-quality, high-quality

214

The case in which the extension is completed. Any application you need does not expose it to any other race.

If you do not have a bug in your browser, you may need to add it to your card. Maintenance cards with storage facilities. We will write a new card.

Make sure you have a clear selection of your latest designs.

Determines the completion of the search prompt

El __

*Personalization*1. Submission:

Muesli (sms. Forms of analysis of mice):

• New mice:

• Social benefits (plan):

*Contracts for job creation: Deal / not Deal 2.*Reflection:

Date: ______________________

Exhibition Post: ______________________________

:Notes: __

3. Posts:

Date: ______________________

Exhibition Post: ______________________________

215

Remarks:

Date: _

Exhibition management: Remarks:

Date:

Exhibition management: Remarks:

Date:

Exhibition management: Remarks:

Date:

Exhibition management: Remarks:

Date:

Exhibition Post: Reproduction: _______

Exercise 75. Watch the Narrow

These are the topics that are most relevant to you and your friends, which you will usually write about and present. We can use your own program for this, which will save the app and set the ability of this feature.

To complete this type of exercise, you can use the form of an extension. In graph GOAL enter, copy, "Select P., which you will find problems with ..." or «Display P. ... or do not write, that's what's going on ».

For each set of options, or to specify a list of values that you want to display or display.

Registration / Release 1:

The window, which is located on either side or side:

1.
2.
3.
4.
5.
6.
7.
8.
9.
10.

Registration / Release 2:

Level, which is used as part of this or displayed: 1.
2. 3. 4. 5. 6. 7.

9. 10.
Registration / Release 3:
Level, which is used as part of this or displayed: 1.
2. 3. 4. 5. 6. 7.
9. 10.

Exercise 76

Create a plan for extending your social contacts.
Create a list of names that include hotels in the area and contact. Please be sure to include it in our specific topic. Distinguish which ones you want to delete.
218
You can permanently edit your list. Shuffle the tag, embed in the progress window.

Name	Plan	Date
1.		
2.		
3.		
4.		
5.		
6.		
7.		
8.		
9.		
10.		

	Plan	Time
1.		
2.		
3.		
4.		
5.		
6.		
7.		
8.		
9.		
10.		

Proofreading77

Schedule your events for the most part, as you will be able to see the latest developments. Distinguish between time and date and complete your plans. You can permanently edit your list.

Exercise 78.
Leibovich test (post-test)

You will need an entry for 24 situations. Some unscrupulous people are aware of the common problems of the day.

Suggest, depending on whether you are in the current situation or whether you have (in the case of a case), a number of cases.

1 - no transport;
2 - light rail;
3 - commuter train;
4 - Intensive travel.

If you want to find out what you are looking for or what you are looking for in a 4-ball location situation:
1 - 0% (0); 2-one (1-33%);
3 - share (34 - 67%);
4 - fixed (68 - 100%).

Troubleshooting

25. Phone coverage of other people's claims. 12 3 4 1234
26. Training in a naughty group. 12 3 4 12 3 4
27. Obed in the chair. 12 3 4 12 3 4
28. Whip coffee in the cafeteria most of the time. 1234 1234
29. Composition of financial statements / statements. 12 3 4 1234
30. Public outreach. 12 3 4 12 3 4
31. Get on the road. 12 3 4 12 3 4
32. Unwrap the work of the other keyhole. 1234 1234
33. Delete entries in postal records. 12 3 4 12 3 4
34. Place a small bowl on the floor. 12 3 4 12 3 4

220

35. Deal with chemistry. 12 3 4 12 3 4
36. The number of people who are not. 12 3 4 12 3 4

37. Attendance of public toilets. 12 3 4 12 3 4
38. Vote in the commune, in which all the pages. 12 3 4 12 3 4
39. Home in the center of women. 12 3 4 12 3 4
40. Without prejudice to the word "submission". 1234 1234
41. Examination of practical or examination materials. 1234 1 234
42. Explain what you do not understand or what you mean by that. 12 3 4 12 3 4
43. Look at the number of people in a glass. 12 3 4 12 3 4
44. Group documents. 12 3 4 12 3 4
45. Engaging in romantic or sexual norms. 1234 1234
46. Load items in a store (with the same number of days). 12 3 4 1234
47. Build a vault. 12 3 4 12 3 4
48. Find a Commercial Agent. 12 3 4 1234

Sell your items in all 24 situations: first item - the value of your items, the value - the level of the situation. Download the most recent results:

Business Rating: ___________________________________

Situation Rating: ___________________________

General image type: ______________________________

Remove your viewers from viewers of the game 4. Divide your search results by:

221

Exercise 79.
Personal test situation
(post-mortem)

Judge the situation, in which case you will find the

most popular sociophobia. This can be a situation where you can get rid of it from a different point of view.

You define situations based on the following principle: "If I cope with these situations and do not experience tension in them, then I will no longer have Secrets of Social phobia." Other languages, do not select situations, which are stored in the window, do not have any names (if any).

Situations that are different in terms of possibilities are very detailed. Other languages, not "create code", and "save to" Belize Orel "are called" and select ". As you can see, we can easily find out about the situation. We also need to find out the specifics, specifics and the best possible situations. If possible, try to find the right one, not the most common one in this situation. It is possible that you will find out what the situations are when completing the challenge 4.

Note that this file does not have a unique situation ("Specify the number of rows and Themes"), as well as which one.

What a great idea:

- Visits to another (as well as to whom?).
- Store this item in a magazine (in which one?).
- Reassignment of the bus stop or at rest.
- Sit in the prime (in which?).
- Serve at a restaurant (as well as with us?).
- Find in the second row of the road (in which? Which?) And all

I would like a rookie.

- Mail the envelope to the mail.
- Whip up a cup of coffee in a coffee shop.
- Execute with a request or a lesson (where? Will I

return?)

• Select in the search box (what? Button?).

222

Increase situations between 1 and 5 numbers.

Let's give you a break, and you'll be welcomed in these situations. For this, use an 8-ball scale, which is 1 - a cocoa-free volley, and 8 - a full panicle. Unleash and recite in the jar the new figure, giving you the support you need. For example, if you are in a situation where you have a bad one, you have "easy disks" (2), or you have a "blue one" (4).

Thank you dear reader person**:**

Regards: Muhammad Bilal

Made in United States
Orlando, FL
24 August 2022

21525638R00096